BREAST CANCER

BREAST CANCER

A Practical Guide to Diagnosis and Treatment

Editor
LOUIS VENET, M.D.

Associate Director, Department of Surgery
Beth Israel Medical Center
and
Professor of Clinical Surgery
Mount Sinai School of Medicine
New York, New York

SP MEDICAL & SCIENTIFIC BOOKS
New York • London

SPECTRUM PUBLICATIONS, INC.

175-20 Wexford Terrace, Jamaica New York

Library of Congress Cataloging in Publication Data

Main entry under title:

Breast cancer.

  Includes index.
  1. Breast—Cancer. I. Venet, Lewis.
[DNLM: 1. Breast neoplasms—Diagnosis. 2. Breast
neoplasms—Therapy. WP870 B8212]
RC280.B8B672   616.9'94'49   79-19357
ISBN 0-89335-102-4

Contributors

ADA B. CHABON, M.D.
Associate Director of Anatomic Pathology
Beth Israel Medical Center
New York, New York
Associate Professor of Clinical Pathology
Mount Sinai School of Medicine
New York, New York

ABRAHAM GEFFEN, M.D.
Attending, Department of Radiology and
    Radiation Therapy
Beth Israel Medical Center
New York, New York
Professor of Clinical Radiology
Mount Sinai School of Medicine
New York, New York

SAUL HOFFMAN, M.D.
Attending, Department of Surgery
Chief, Section of Plastic Surgery
Beth Israel Medical Center
New York, New York
Clinical Professor of Surgery
Mount Sinai School of Medicine
New York, New York

BERNARD KABAKOW, M.D.
Attending Physician in charge of Medical
    Oncology
Beth Israel Medical Center
New York, New York
Associate Clinical Professor of Medicine
Mount Sinai School of Medicine
New York, New York

MAX NEEDLEMAN, M.D.
Attending, Department of Psychiatry
Beth Israel Medical Center
New York, New York
Associate Clinical Professor Emeritus of
    Psychiatry
Mount Sinai School of Medicine
New York, New York

MYRON P. NOBLER, M.D.
Attending, Department of Radiology and
    Radiation Therapy
Chief of Radiation Therapy
Beth Israel Medical Center
New York, New York
Associate Professor of Radiotherapy
Mount Sinai School of Medicine
New York, New York

PETER I. PRESSMAN, M.D.
Attending, Department of Surgery
Beth Israel Medical Center
New York, New York
Clinical Consultant, Guttman Institute
New York, New York
Associate Clinical Professor of Surgery
Mount Sinai School of Medicine
New York, New York

PHILIP STRAX, M.D.
Medical Director, Guttman Institute
New York, New York
Director of Radiology
LaGuardia Hospital
Forest Hills, New York
Associate Clinical Professor of Community
    and Preventive Medicine
New York Medical College
New York, New York

NATALIE STRUTYNSKY, M.D.
Associate Attending, Department of
    Radiology and Radiation Therapy
Beth Israel Medical Center
New York, New York
Assistant Professor of Radiology
Mount Sinai School of Medicine
New York, New York

LOUIS VENET, M.D.
Associate Director, Department of Surgery
Chief, Section of Breast Surgery

Beth Israel Medical Center
New York, New York
Professor of Clinical Surgery
Mount Sinai School of Medicine
New York, New York

ROBERT C. WALLACH, M.D.
Director of Obstetrics and Gynecology
Beth Israel Medical Center
New York, New York
Professor of Clinical Obstetrics and
    Gynecology
Mount Sinai School of Medicine
New York, New York

Foreword

In the practice of medicine today, patients with carcinoma of the breast are among the most difficult challenges faced by the profession. The causes of this difficulty are many; but perhaps the most important are related to the unpredictable biologic behavior of these tumors. Examples of this unique behavior include its propensity to occur in all decades of adulthood, to cause death in a matter of months in some patients while in others to peacefully coexist for years, and to apparently respond in certain instances to therapeutic modalities as diverse as surgery, hormonal manipulation and radiotherapy.

The unpredictable nature of carcinoma of the breast has spawned many controversies concerning its management. Short-term claims of success have all too often evaporated into unpublished long-term failures. Claims and counter-claims based on too few clinical observations over short periods of time have resulted in confusion in the minds of physicians, both specialist and generalist. This controversy, expressed in both the scientific as well as lay press, has caused untold difficulty as well to patients with breast tumors.

Patients with mass lesions of the breast are often well versed in the therapeutic options available to them as well as the reported results of certain authors and clinics. Indeed their knowledge of the subject could be envied by some of our students. All too often, however, this knowledge lacks the scientific detachment and discrimination necessary to formulate a sound program of management. It is disheartening to the practitioner to consult with patients who have already decided on their therapeutic program and are seeking not counsel but a cooperative therapist. The temptation to reject these patients must be resisted since their conflicts are often mirrors of our own ambiguity.

How then is the physician expected to respond to the concerns and needs of his patients with carcinoma of the breast? This text has been written in an effort to provide the practitioner with answers to this question which are both practical and comprehensive. The summation of the individual chapters is the total management of the patient with carcinoma of the breast. This book also represents the clinical experiences of a group of specialists actively collaborating on a daily basis. With one exception, all are members of the staff of the Beth Israel Medical Center. The content of the text is derived in large measure from a yearly symposium "The Management of Breast Carcinoma" sponsored by Beth Israel. This symposium by all criteria is one of our most successful educational efforts.

The task of the editor of a multi-authored text is to synthesize in an orderly and logical manner the information which is provided the reader. On occasion, he must also mediate and reconcile divergent recommendations. With carcinoma of the breast, Dr. Louis Venet is eminently qualified for the task. From a career which has been devoted to all phases of this subject, he brings a wealth of knowledge and experience which is reflected in the high standard of excellence which has been achieved by this text. As a result of his achievements in the early detection of breast cancer, Dr. Venet has participated in numerous scientific projects designed to improve the care of these patients. He is therefore capable of evaluating and presenting those aspects of therapy which have had meaningful impact on both the physical and psychologic well-being of patients with carcinoma of the breast.

Charles K. McSherry, M.D.
Director of Surgery
Beth Israel Medical Center
Professor of Surgery
Mount Sinai School of Medicine

Preface

This book has been written as a result of the annual Breast Cancer Conferences sponsored by the Beth Israel Medical Center in affiliation with the Page and William Black Post-Graduate School of Medicine of the Mount Sinai School of Medicine and the New York City Division of the American Cancer Society. At the time of this writing the 5th Annual Conference has been completed, and another is scheduled for next year. These programs have received favorable responses and there have been repeated suggestions to me, as program chairman, that conference proceedings be published as such. My colleagues and I considered this possibility and unanimously decided to enlarge upon the individual and panel presentations by preparing chapters with information presented in much greater detail and depth.

Each chapter is written by an individual with considerable experience in his or her chosen field. They have all contributed over the years to the annual program, and with the exception of Dr. Philip Strax, are all staff members of the Beth Israel Medical Center. The opinions expressed are those of the individual authors, with some editorial suggestions relating to content and, or, mode of presentation. They do not represent the official opinions of the Beth Israel Medical Center, the Mount Sinai School of Medicine or of any other organization.

This book is not intended to be an exhaustive treatise on all aspects of breast cancer. Rather, the purpose is to present the viewpoints of clinicians of various disciplines who are involved with the management of patients with breast tumors. Such patients require a multidisciplinary approach to their care. We are in a new and rapidly changing era with regard to all aspects of the management of patients with potential or actual breast cancer. No longer is the surgeon the only caretaker. In the past 10-15 years, there has been a rapid development and rise in the use of mammography, and a better understanding of the histopathology of breast cancer. In addition, there has been great emphasis on the education of the public about cancer in general, and breast cancer in particular. Surgeons have had to alter their approaches to treatment. Many patients arrive at the surgeon's office with a minimal tumor detected by periodic self-examination, or by clinical or radiographic screening. Surgeons make recommendations about treatment, but often second opinions and consultations are obtained. The decision regarding therapy is not necessarily individual, but is frequently collective, since radiologists, oncologists, plastic surgeons, pathologists, radiation therapists, psychiatrists, gynecologists, family physicians and the patient herself and her family may be involved in the decision-making process. Thus, the reader of this volume may note some differences of approach by the various collaborators. However, in actual clinical practice, these differences are usually resolved after consultations amongst members of the "Team". A flexible approach to management is necessary in order to select the mode of therapy best suited for the individual patient's psychosocial requirements and the physical aspects of her breast cancer.

In the first chapter, Dr. Strutynsky develops the basics of mammography. Obviously, one cannot learn to be a mammographer simply by reading this chapter. However, all physicians and others involved in the care of breast cancer patients should have some basic knowledge of the advantages and limitations of this diagnostic technique. At the present time, because of the controversy about the use of mammography, many patients, by avoiding mammography may lose the best opportunity for the early detection of breast cancer. It is because of the importance of mammography and the concern of many about the radiogenic risks, that Dr. Abraham Geffen has devoted an entire chapter to the risks versus benefits of mammography. At the national level, a great deal of interest and effort is apparent in the attempt to obtain more information on this issue. It is probable that data from the breast cancer demonstration centers supported by the National Cancer Institute and the American Cancer Society will help to resolve some of these issues in the future.

In a second chapter, Dr. Geffen has reviewed the problem of radionucleotide scanning in the management of patients with breast cancer. This is also a controversial subject since there is, at present, no unanimity regarding when, and what area to scan,—or not to scan.

I consider Dr. Philip Strax a member of the Beth Israel Medical Center family since we have been associated together in the so-called "H.I.P." mammography study since 1962. He has become identified as the person most knowledgeable and most enthusiastic about screening for breast cancer. He has been invited to present his viewpoints at conferences throughout the world and is eminently qualified to render the overview of the present status of screening.

Dr. Robert Wallach, a gynecologist, insists that his staff examine the breasts as part of the routine "gyn" exam. The gynecologist is often the first person from whom the patient seeks advice regarding breast problems. He or she must therefore be very well informed about breast diseases and should be expert in the examination of the breasts. Dr. Wallach discusses these aspects in his chapter.

Dr. Max Needleman has been called in consultation for patients with breast diseases on numerous occasions. He has had considerable experience with patients both before and after mastectomy. I have personally found his advice and support of great assistance in carrying patients through the experience of approaching surgery and of coping with the impact of having breast cancer. The psychosomatic aspects of breast cancer are receiving well-deserved attention in the medical literature, and Dr. Needleman adds some provocative viewpoints in his chapter.

The final diagnosis of breast cancer must be made by the pathologist. However, as a result of the increasing use of mammography and the detection of minimal lesions, the pathologist is approaching the histologic area where the boundary line between a benign and malignant lesion is not clear cut. Dr. deChabon discusses this and other problems relating to pathology in her chapter.

Surgery has been the primary mode of therapy in the past, and still maintains a high order of importance. Dr. Peter Pressman has devoted himself to the care of patients with breast cancer and has contributed to the literature on this subject. The standard Halsted radical mastectomy was the operation performed routinely in this country 10-15 years ago. However, at present the surgeon has many operations that are being advocated both in the medical and lay literature. Dr. Pressman presents his viewpoints in a logical manner based upon his own experience and his extensive knowledge of the literature.

In the past, radiation therapy was considered an adjunct to surgery. It was used primarily to supplement surgery in advanced cases or as a last resort when surgery was considered ineffective. However, particularly with the availability of modern equipment and technology there are increasing reports in which radiation therapy is recommended for the primary treatment of breast cancer. Dr. Nobler has been utilizing this approach and discusses this and other aspects of radiation therapy in his chapter.

A great deal of attention and enthusiasm is apparent with regard to the possibilities of reconstruction of the breast following mastectomy. This field of surgery is changing rapidly, but enough experience has been obtained to indicate that reconstruction is possible with excellent results. Dr. Saul Hoffman devotes his chapter to a review of the present status of reconstruction of the breast.

The final chapter has been written by Dr. Bernard Kabakow, an internist and oncologist. This specialty has assumed rapidly increasing importance in the care of cancer patients. The oncologist is now assuming a major, and often, the major role in the care of breast cancer patients. Chemotherapy, hormone therapy, immunotherapy are all modalities which fall most naturally into the province of the oncologist. In addition, the family physician, internist or oncologist is often the "captain of the Team" and follows the patient through all phases of her disease. Dr. Kabakow presents a detailed discussion of the medical management of patients with breast cancer.

I wish to express my appreciation for the continuing support, enthusiasm, and cooperation of my colleagues who have contributed the chapters to this book. Mrs. Stephanie Castrovinci has been of invaluable assistance, and for this I am deeply grateful. The publisher, Mr. Maurice Ancharoff, and his Managing Editor Mrs. Anita Steinberg, have been most helpful in the technical aspects of the preparation of this volume.

Louis Venet, M.D.
May, 1979

Contents

CHAPTER 1

Mammography

NATALIE STRUTYNSKY

HISTORICAL BACKGROUND

The history of mammography, or the radiographic examination of the breasts, is surprisingly brief and goes back only 40 years. The earliest examinations were attempted in the 1920s and 1930s; however, the results were unsatisfactory because of inadequate soft tissue technique. The French investigator Leborgne (Leborgne, 1951), in the 1940s, was the first to achieve sufficient details on mammograms to visualize fine calcifications in breast cancers. In the U.S., the great pioneers in mammography were Gershon-Cohen and Egan. In their classic publications in the 1950s and 1960s the basics of diagnostic mammography were established, (Gershon-Cohen et al., 1960; Gershon-Cohen et al., 1953; Gershon-Cohen et al., 1966; Egan, 1969; Egan, 1964; Egan, 1960)

The technical aspects of mammography are relatively simple: each breast is exposed to ionizing radiation (x-rays), using soft tissue technique—i.e., low kilovoltage in the range of 28 kvp to 38 kvp. A highly sensitive x-ray film, packed in a vacuum cassette, is used to achieve optimum diagnostic detail. A specialized mammography machine is usually necessary to provide an exact output at this low kilovoltage level while delivering the least possible radiation dose to the breast. A minimum of two views (cranio-caudad and lateral) of each breast are taken; additional views may be added in some cases.

Xeromammography also uses an x-ray beam to produce the diganostic image of the breast, however, instead of the x-ray film a selenium-coated aluminum plate is used to record the diagnostic image. This image is then transferred to a sheet of white plastic-coated paper which represents the final diagnostic record. Wolfe (Wolfe, 1968; Wolfe, 1967) is well-known for his work with xeromammography in the U.S. and he remains one of the chief proponents of this method. The over-all diagnostic accuracy of the two methods is quite similar, although as might be expected, proponents of each method have claimed superiority!

There are several advantages and disadvantages that are associated with each system. The important ones and those relevant to this chapter are:

a) The cost of renting xerographic equipment has become prohibitive for many radiological practices.

b) The radiation dosage is *lower* with the newest low-dose and rare earth screens and films than it is with xero-mammography. This is an extremely important factor in view of the current concern with radiation exposure. (Factors a and b are largely responsible for the preference of film mammography over xeromammography by most radiologists today.)

c) One of the great advantages of xero-mammography (as it pertains to this chapter) is the ease of photographic reproduction and the great clarity of the images. (For this reason all the illustrations in this chapter will be drawn from xero-mammographic material.)

There is one important difference between film and xerographic images that must be understood before studying the illustrations. The xerographic image is a photographic *positive* image, as opposed to the negative one on the x-ray film. Therefore, high density structures such as bones and calcium will appear dark on xerograms while they are white on the x-ray film.

THE NORMAL BREAST

The radiographic appearance of the breast varies according to the age, parity, and even the menstrual cycle of the woman. It is, therefore, important to review the changes in the breast during these various phases in order to understand their effects on the diganostic quality of the mammogram.

The normal breast is composed of 15 to 20 lobes, each one with its own secretory duct emptying into the nipple. The main ducts subdivide in the periphery of the breast and eventually terminate in multiple lobules, where the secretory cells are located. A loose connective tissue stroma is interspersed with the epithelial elements; thicker connective tissue strands form the suspensory ligaments of the breast. In Figure 1 a lateral mammogram of a 12-year-old pubertal girl shows developing breast tissue. The linear structures that can be seen extending from the areola posteriorly are a combination of proliferating ducts as well the supporting connective tissue stroma. The breast is not yet fully developed, and some radiolucent fat can be seen interspersed with the denser parenchyma and stroma. A clear radiolucent fat-line can be identified; this separates the developing breast tissue from the pectoral muscles.

Figure 2 shows the radiographic appearance of a normal 18-year-old nulliparous young woman in whom the development of breast tissue is com-

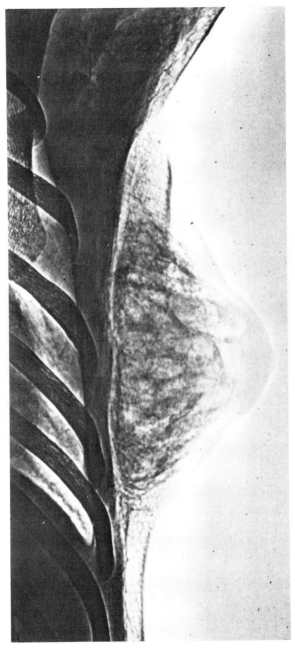

Fig. 1. Lateral view of the developing breast in a 12-year-old girl. The breast shows a mottled radiographic appearance due to a mixture of fat and parenchyma. Note the black appearance of the ribs on xerography.

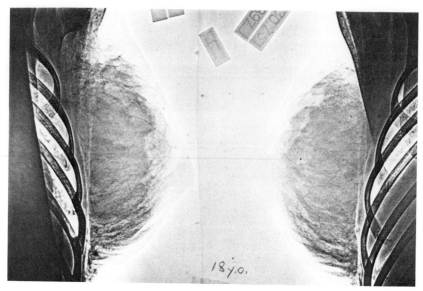

Fig. 2. Lateral views of both breasts of a nulliparous 18-year-old young woman. The breasts appear markedly dense due to the absence of any significant amount of fat in the parenchyma.

plete. The breasts show a homogeneous, dense appearance, and it is impossible to identify discrete structures such as main ducts. There is some subcutaneous fat identified as a radiolucent area underneath the skin; otherwise the breast lacks any significant fat content. The retromammary space can be seen separating breast from pectoral muscles. The curvilinear densities that traverse the breast on both sides are blood vessels and supporting ligaments.

After pregnancy a marked involution of the parenchymal and stromal elements of the breast takes place and considerable replacement with fatty tissue occurs. Note the striking difference from Figures 1 and 2 in the radiographic appearance of the breast shown in Figure 3. This woman is 24 years old and has borne one child. The breast has a pronounced translucent appearance so that small structures such as ducts, small vessels, and ligaments can be identified. It is this radiolucent quality of the intra-mammary fat which enables us to identify even very small tumors with a high degree of accuracy. In contrast, examination of the very dense image of the breast shown in Figure 2 will be likely to yield the lowest degree of accuracy.

With further advancing age there is even more involution of both the parenchymal and stromal elements of the breast. A typical mammogram of a post-menopausal woman is shown in Figure 4. There is almost complete

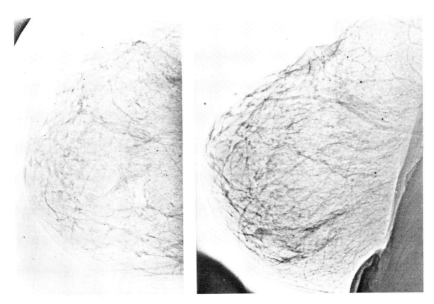

Fig. 3. Cranio-caudad and lateral views of the breast of a 24-year-old woman who has borne one child. The difference from the breast of a nulliparous woman is striking because of the marked replacement of breast parenchyma by fat.

replacement of the entire breast by fat. Some ducts are seen close to the areola, and vessels can be identified clearly. A frequent finding in elderly women is arterial calcification. The dark, wavy structures traversing the breast in this view are calcified arterioles. Note the extremely sharp delineation of the calcium on this image. This is caused by the edge-enhancement effect of the xerographic process—one of the significant advantages of xero-mammography in the diagnosis of abnormal breast calcifications.

MAMMARY DYSPLASIA

The normal changes in the appearance of the breast, as described above, will not occur in women who remain nulliparous or who develop mammary dysplasia. This term has been accepted to include a broad group of histological changes in the breast in which there is an imbalanced proportion of supporting connective tissue and parenchyma as well as an over-proliferation of both. The exact etiology of this imbalance is not known, but it is thought to be produced by a hormonal dysfunction (Golinger, 1978).

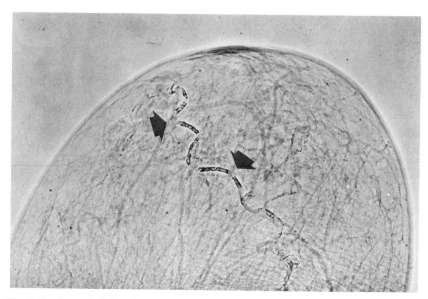

Fig. 4. Carnio-caudad view showing the typical, fatty breast of a post-menopausal patient. The black wavy structure (arrows) is a calcified arteriole. Note the black appearance of calcium on xerography.

The pathological changes of mammary dysplasia include a wide spectrum of abnormalities such as ductal proliferation, cyst formation, proliferation of the terminal ductules and lobules, as well as an excess of connective tissue. Except for the gross fibro-cystic changes, the individual histologic abnormalities correlate poorly with the radiographic appearance in women known to have mammary dysplasia. For this reason it is best not to attempt a specific histologic diagnosis, such as adenosis or ductal hyperplasia, on the basis of the x-ray appearance of the breast, but instead to use the inclusive term mammary dysplasia in making the diagnosis.

In Figure 5 we see the mammogram of a 36-year-old woman, para O, who presents with the complaint of pain in both breasts and multiple lumps on physical examination. The radiographic appearance would best be described as an inhomogeneous breast with alternating areas of radiolucency and density. The histology report on the biopsy of such a breast will include the whole spectrum of manifestations of mammary dysplasia such as cystic changes, ductal hyperplasia, adenosis, and fibrosis.

Figures 6 and 7 show mammograms in which multiple, tortuous, linear densities extend from the nipple into the parenchyma of the breasts. This appearance illustrates the "prominent ductal pattern" that has been de-

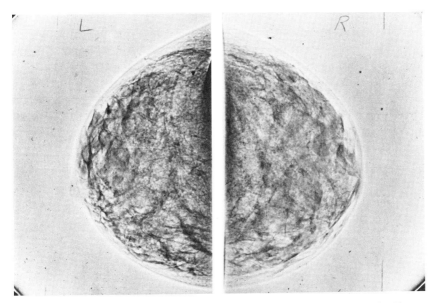

Fig. 5. Cranio-caudad views of both breasts of a patient with mammary dysplasia. The inhomogeneous or mottled appearance of the breast is very similar in appearance to the breast of a young, developing or nulliparous woman (Fig. 1).

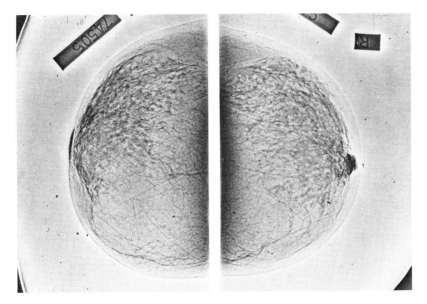

Fig. 6. Carnio-caudad views of both breasts with a prominent ductal pattern. Note the tortuous, linear densities extending from the nipples into at least half of the parenchyma.

scribed by Wolfe (Wolfe, 1976). According to his work, women with this
type of mammary dysplasia are more likely to develop breast cancer than
are women having breast parenchyma patterns in other categories. The his-
tologic-radiographic correlation is based on true ductal hyperplasia as well
as on periductal collagenosis.

An important diagnostic feature that is seen in all these examples of
mammary dysplasia (Figures 5-7) is the striking symmetry in the degree of
involvement of the two breasts. This symmetry is seen in almost all cases of
mammary dysplasia.

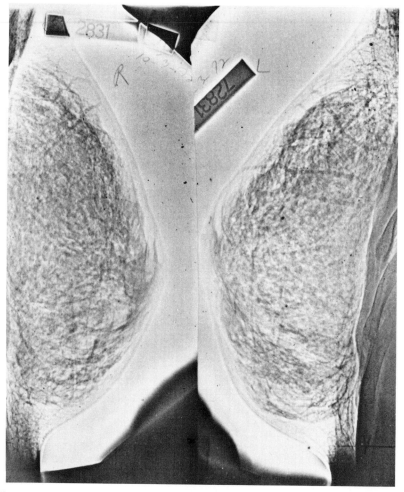

Fig. 7. Lateral views of both breasts of a patient with severe mammary dysplasia. The
prominent ductal pattern involves every portion of each breast. Note the striking symmetry
of involvement of the two breasts.

In the next illustration, Figure 8, there are multiple large, oval and round masses present in both breasts. Some of the masses are confluent; in other areas discrete borders can be delineated. This appearance is usually caused by the presence of multiple large and small cysts. However, even in this case the biopsy will usually show all the other components of mammary dysplasia.

The least common form of mammary dysplasia is pure fibrosis. This is illustrated in Figure 9, in which a homogeneous density can be seen in the upper half of the left breast. The involvement in this patient is exceptionally asymmetric. On biopsy, pure fibrosis was found with no accompanying ductal abnormalities.

BENIGN MASSES OF THE BREAST

Sometimes a patient presents with a single dominant cyst in one breast without the clinical or radiographic evidence of dysplasia in the contralateral breast. In Figure 10 a large, oval mass is seen in the upper half of the breast. A clearly defined border can be seen anteriorly and superiorly, the surrounding parenchyma is slightly displaced by this mass. The largest diameter of the mass is oriented along the direction of the supporting ligaments. This is a characteristic radiographic appearance of a large cyst without any accompanying dysplasia in the remaining portions of the breast.

An almost identical radiographic appearance is seen in the mammogram (Figure 11) of another patient. A spherical mass is present just inferior to the nipple. The borders of the mass are clearly demarcated, and there is a halo of radiolucent fat around the lesion. The surrounding parenchyma is minimally compressed. This is the typical appearance of a fibroadenoma, the most common benign tumor encountered in the breast.

The age distribution for the development of cysts and for that of fibro-adenomas is different: Cysts are common among women from 35 to 45 years old, while fibroadenomas occur in younger women, with a peak incidence at approximately 25 years of age. The two lesions differ somewhat on clinical palpation; a needle aspiration will usually establish the diagnosis of cyst. Radiographically, however, the appearances can be identical. The only radiographic feature which is pathognomonic of a fibroadenoma is the coarse, heavy calcification in a degenerated fibroadenoma.

In Figure 12 a dense, round calcification is seen in the breast. There is an area of marked halo formation around the calcification due to the physical property of edge-enhancement of xerography. The soft tissue component of the fibroadenoma is not visible in this case, as it is masked by the density of the dysplastic breast. This type of calcification is quite specific and diagnos-

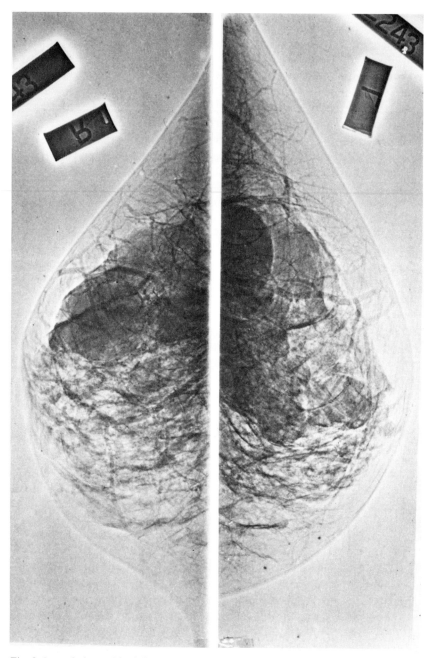

Fig. 8. Lateral views of both breasts in a patient with fibrocystic disease. Note the smooth, convex borders of multiple large and small cysts. The left breast is more severely involved than the right.

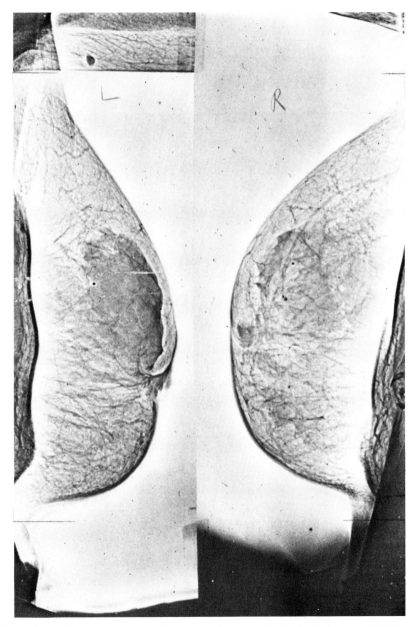

Fig. 9. Lateral mammograms showing an area of non-specific density in the upper half of the left breast. Pure fibrosis was found on biopsy of that area.

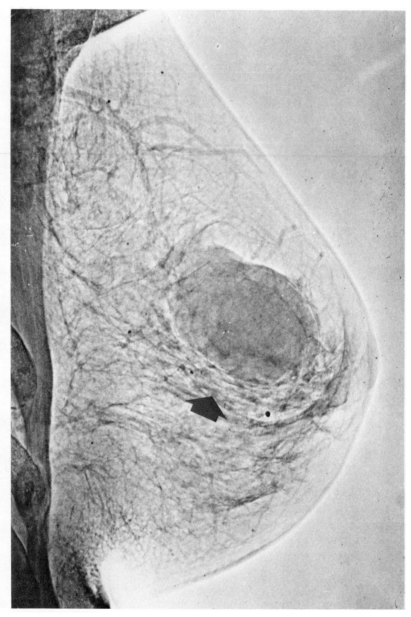

Fig. 10. Lateral mammogram showing a single large cyst in an otherwise normal breast. Note the smooth borders anteriorly and superiorly and the concave appearance of displaced breast structures (arrow) below the inferior margin of the cyst.

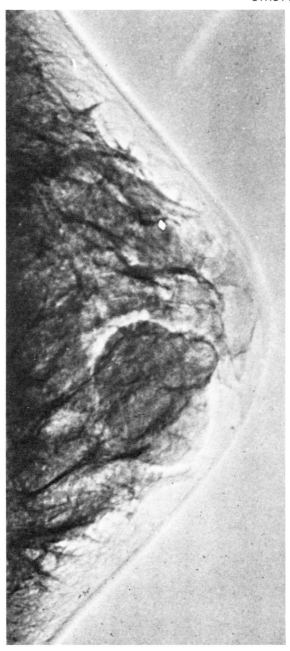

Fig. 11. Lateral mammogram of a young girl with a fibroadenoma seen just inferior to the nipple. The margins of the tumor are smooth and well demarcated. The white halo of compressed fat around the tumor is typical of a fibroadenoma.

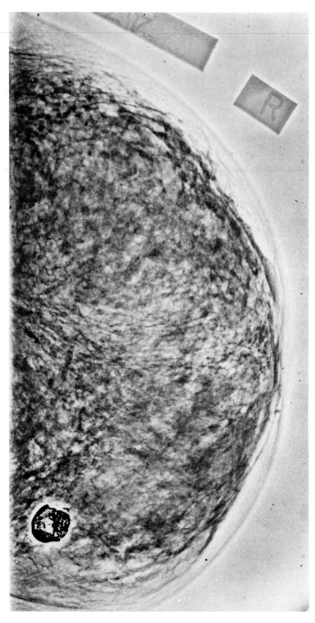

Fig. 12. Lateral mammogram showing a calcified fibroadenoma near the inferior skin fold in a markedly dysplastic breast. The calcification is coarse, large, and round in contour. The marked white halo around the calcification is due to the physical property of edge-enhancement of xerography.

tic of a fibroadenoma. In approximately 10% to 15% of cases fibroadenomas are multiple and/or bilateral.

An intraductal papilloma is a lesion frequently associated with nipple discharge or bleeding. Most of these tumors are small and cannot be identified on mammograms. Occasionally a tumor grows to such an extent that it produces a visible bulge in the duct that can be seen on a mammogram. In Figure 13, in the left breast, there is a single linear, somewhat wavy density that extends from the nipple posteriorly. No similar structure can be identified in the contralateral breast. This density represents a large papilloma growing in and dilating one of the major ducts. There is usually no calcification associated with these tumors; rarely they may be bilateral.

Lipomas are found frequently in the breast, which is not surprising considering the large fat content of the breast. Many breast biopsies could be misdiagnosed as lipomas. However, a diagnosis of lipoma should be reserved for those patients whose mammograms show a true fibrous capsule around the fatty content. A typical lipoma is shown in Figure 14, in the lower half of the breast. The entire mass is radiolucent; the thin curvilinear density surrounding the mass is the fibrous capsule. Clinically, these tumors are frequently mistaken for large cysts because of the soft, or "cystic," consistency on palpation.

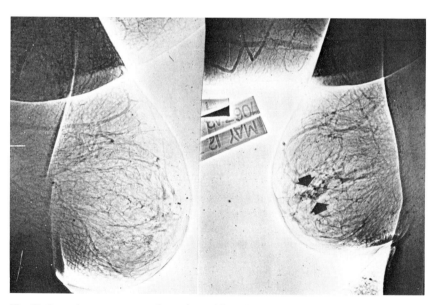

Fig. 13. Lateral mammograms of a patient with an intraductal papilloma in the left breast. Note the typical ribbon- like density (arrows) which extends from the nipple posteriorly. The location of the tumor in a major duct is also characteristic.

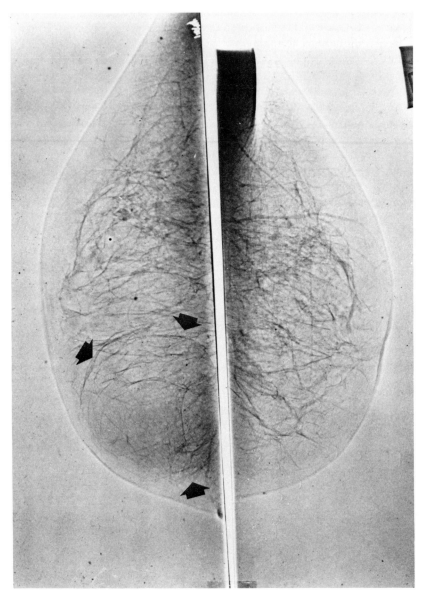

Fig. 14. Lateral mammogram showing a lipoma in the right breast (arrows). The circular fine line is the fibrous capsule. The tumor itself is indistinguishable from the rest of the fat in the breast.

Various other benign tumors occur in the breast, although much less frequently than the tumors described above. Almost all of the benign mesenchymal tumors have been found in the breast, including fibromas, neurofibromas, vascular tumors, etc. The epithelial elements can give rise to sweat gland tumors. The radiographic appearance of these tumors is nonspecific, the final diagnosis depending on the histologic interpretation.

BREAST CANCER

The radiographic signs of breast cancer are subdivided into two categories—primary and secondary. The two major primary signs of breast malignancy include the presence of a mass with certain radiographic features of malignancy and the presence of malignant tumor calcifications. A third primary sign has been added by Wolfe (Wolfe, 1967)—a segmental prominent duct pattern in the breast.

The secondary signs of malignancy include increased vascularity of the breast, skin changes, retraction of the nipple, and the presence of axillary lymphadenopathy. All of these signs are summarized in Table I.

Table I.
Primary and Secondary Signs of Breast Cancer

Primary	Secondary
1. Presence of mass with malignant features	1. Increased vascularity of breast
2. Presence of tumor micro-calcifications	2. Skin edema
3. Segmental ductal prominence in one breast	3. Skin retraction
	4. Nipple retraction
	5. Axillary lymphadenopathy

The characteristic radiographic feature of a malignant mass is markedly irregular, knobby, poorly defined contour, as opposed to the smooth, well delineated contour of a benign lesion. This malignant feature is demonstrated in Figure 15. The mass is located in the upper half of the breast, close to the chest wall. The irregular, knobby border is striking over the anterior aspect of the mass.

Another characteristic appearance of a malignant breast lesion is shown in Figure 16. In addition to the dense nodule in the central portion of the breast, there are innumerable linear extensions radiating from the nodule into the surrounding breast parenchyma. These extensions give the tumor a

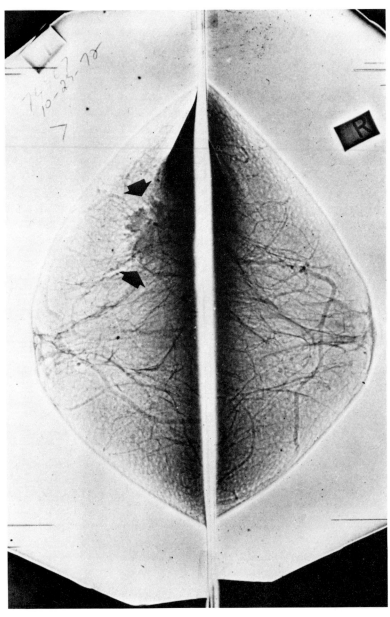

Fig. 15. Lateral mammogram revealing a cancer in the left breast (arrows). The tumor outline is very irregular in contrast to the smooth contours of a benign lesion.

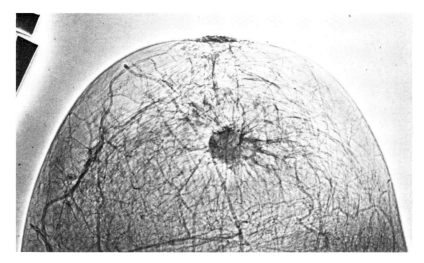

Fig. 16. Typical appearance of a scirrhous breast cancer. Note the linear extensions from the periphery of the tumor nodule, which give this lesion a spiculated or stellate appearance.

spiculated or stellate appearance. Careful pathologic study has shown that these linear extensions represent tumor infiltration along breast lymphatics, along ducts, and along fibrous ligaments. It has also been shown that a considerable portion of the linear structures are a desmoplastic fibrotic reaction in the breast, stimulated by the tumor. The desmoplastic reaction around the tumor is responsible for the discrepancy in the size of the tumor as seen on mammograms and as palpated by the clinician. The mass always appears much larger on physical examination, since the fibrous reaction around the tumor is indistinguishable from the tumor itself.

Sometimes the carcinoma does not have the typical spiculated or knobby appearance but presents only as an area of increased density in one breast. This is illustrated in Figure 17, in which an area of poorly demarcated density in the lower half of the left breast is the only clue to the presence of an abnormality. This appearance is seen in cases of lobular cancer. It should be noted that in a breast with a marked degree of mammary dysplasia (i.e., having a very dense radiographic appearance), this type of cancer will be completely hidden.

The segmental or localized prominent ductal pattern, which has been described by Wolfe (Wolfe, 1967) as a primary sign of breast cancer, depends on the periductal collagen deposition that occurs with some intraductal carcinomas. The tumor itself may contribute very little to the density and prominence of the ducts. The segmental, or localized, prominence of ducts should not be confused with the generalized prominent ductal pattern,

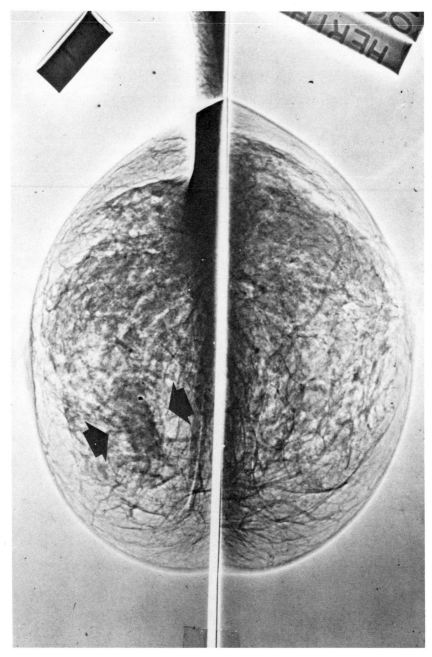

Fig. 17. Lateral views of both breasts. Note the area of assymetrical increased density in the left breast (arrows). This may be the only finding in some cases of lobular cancer.

which involves both breasts symmetrically and is a form of severe mammary dysplasia. According to Wolfe's work, patients in whom localized segmental ductal prominence is found in one breast only, the incidence of cancer will be about 40%.

The other major sign of breast cancer is the presence of tumor calcifications. The characteristic appearance of the calcifications has been described as multiple, small, punctate calcium deposits clustered closely together in one area of the breast. The significance of the number of calcifications was studied by Rogers and Powell (Rogers et al., 1972). In a series of 72 biopsy-proven cases, the authors found that among patients who had 15 or more microcalcifications in an area 1cm^2 of the breast, the malignancy rate was 82%. Among patients with 6 to 16 microcalcifications, the incidence of cancer was 23%. No cancer was found on the basis of microcalcifications alone in patients with five or fewer calcifications per 1 cm^2 area of the breast.

The size of calcifications varies from very small, barely visible to fairly large deposits (up to 1 mm in diameter), but it almost never reaches the size identified in benign intraductal concretions or in fibroadenomas. The shape of calcifications also varies from fairly smooth round contours to bizarre, pleomorphic shapes. Figure 18 shows the typical appearance of clustered tumor calcifications in a breast cancer. In this case there is an associated stellate appearance to the tumor as well. The number of calcifications is certainly more than 15 per 1 cm^2 area; the calcifications are all closely packed into one small area of the breast. Compare these to the benign intraductal calcifications due to secretory disease, which are shown in Figure 19. The benign calcifications have a smooth, rod-shaped or branching appearance; they often are round in shape when seen end-on. They tend to be uniform and fairly large in size and are evenly distributed throughout the breast. Frequently they can be seen in both breasts symmetrically.

In Figure 20 the tumor calcifications are seen throughout the entire breast. The small size of the calcifications as well as the closely packed clustering are typical of malignancy, although the extent of involvement of the breast is unusual. In spite of this extensive disease, the patient did not have any palpable masses and presented clinically with Paget's disease of the nipple. Biopsy and subsequent mastectomy showed an extensive comedocarcinoma of the entire breast. Many axillary nodes were also positive for malignancy.

It must be emphasized that these tiny tumor calcifications can pinpoint a small cancer of the breast while the tumor is still subclinical and completely undiagnosable by any other means. Many of these cases will be diagnosed at an early stage of the disease before metastases to nodes or other sites occur. The early identification of these small cancers is one of the major benefits of routine screening by mammography of asymptomatic women.

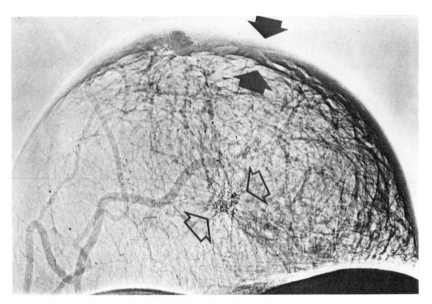

Fig. 18. Typical appearance of malignant calcifications (lower arrows). Note the close clustering of the tiny calcific densities, which appear dark on xerograms. The marked increase in skin thickness (top arrows) as well as increased vascularity are both secondary signs of breast malignancy, which are present in this case.

The secondary signs of breast cancer include skin edema, skin retraction, nipple retraction, increased vascularity of the breast, and the presence of axillary adenopathy. Several of these signs can be seen in Figure 18 (in addition to the primary signs of spiculated mass and tumor calcifications). The most strking finding in this case is the marked increase in skin thickness overlying the breast. The skin thickness as seen on normal mammograms is usually 1 mm to 2 mm, and in this patient the thickest part measured 2 cm! This finding is attributed to lymphatic plugging by the tumor with resultant edema of the skin. Another secondary sign present in this example is the marked increase in the size and number of veins in the involved breast.

Skin retraction, or skin puckering, also a secondary sign of malignancy, is shown in Figure 21. The normal smooth, convex curve of the skin outline is interrupted in the upper half of the breast over a small infiltrating cancer. Old sugical scars frequently mimic this appearance in a patient with previous breast surgery.

Unfortunately there is a group of breast cancers that lack all the specific characteristics of malignancy as described above. The radiographic appearance of these cancers is often identical to that of a benign fibroadenoma or cyst. The tumors in this category are medullary cancer, intracystic cancer,

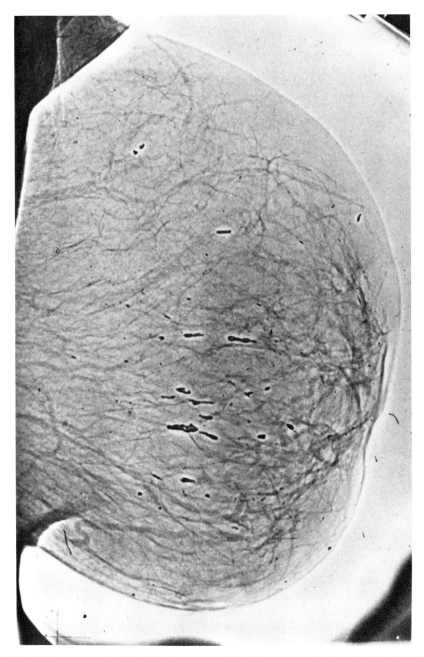

Fig. 19. Benign intraductal calcifications are scattered throughout the breast in this lateral view. Note the rod-shaped, smooth appearance and the fairly large size.

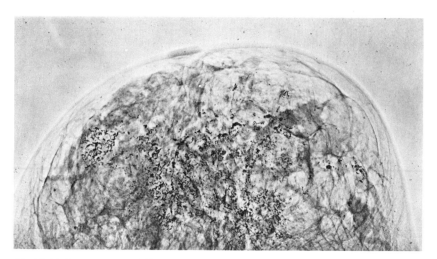

Fig. 20. Malignant tumor calcifications are seen in all parts of this breast. This case illustrates the bizarre shapes and the variety of sizes of carcinomatous calcifications.

and a few other histologic types. The case illustrated in Figure 22 shows a large mass in the inferior half of the right breast. The mass has well delineated, sharp borders and shows no evidence of invasion of the surrounding breast parenchyma. There are no tumor calcifications in this mass, and no secondary signs of cancer can be detected in the breast. At surgery this tumor proved to be an intrasystic carcinoma—i.e. a carcinoma arising inside an ordinary breast cyst. The safest clinical course to follow would be excision of any dominant mass regardless of the radiographic features. One might ask then, if every lump is going to be biopsied, why bother with mammography? The following case presentations will illustrate some of the reasons mammography should be performed.

INDICATIONS FOR MAMMOGRAPHY

The patient whose mammogram is shown in Figure 23 presented with a clinically obvious large cancer in the right breast. On physical examination and on mammography gross nipple retraction was seen. The planned course of treatment was breast biopsy followed by mastectomy on the right side. However, mammography revealed a small stellate lesion in the clinically normal left breast. Both lesions were found to be malignant at biopsy and a bilateral mastectomy was performed. Approximately 1% to 4% of

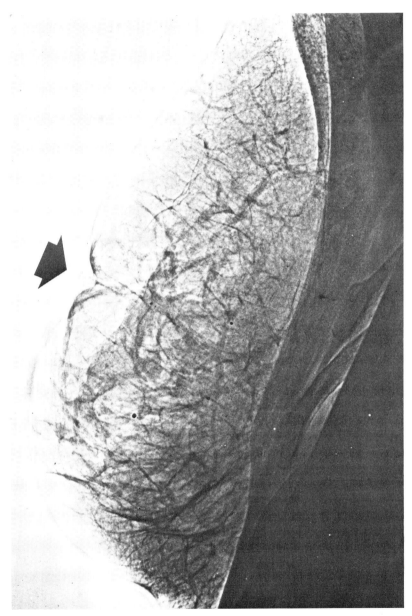

Fig. 21. Skin dimpling (arrow) over a small infiltrating cancer of the breast. Tumor infiltration along fibrous septa and retraction of the septa results in this appearance.

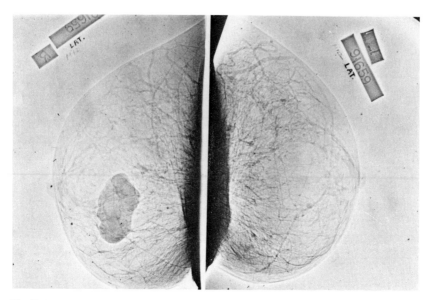

Fig. 22. Large mass in right breast has well delineated borders and looks deceptively benign.
This lesion is a large cyst with a carcinoma arising from the inside epithelial lining of the cyst.

breast cancers will be bilateral at the time of diagnosis; a somewhat higher
percentage of patients will develop a cancer in the second breast post-mastectomy. The diagnosis of breast cancer in one breast is therefore an indication for routine baseline and follow-up mammography of the other breast.

The patient whose mammogram is shown in Figure 24 was admitted for
surgery on the right breast for a mass near the inframammary fold. Clinically, the lesion was thought to be benign, probably a fibroadenoma. However, the mammogram disclosed an unsuspected stellate lesion in the upper
half of the same breast. The clinically obvious benign nodule was, in fact,
benign. However, the unsuspected lesion was a cancer. Thus, even in a
breast with an obvious lump a second unsuspected cancer can coexist.

At this point it would be useful to summarize and tabulate the currently
acceptable indications for mammography (Table II, modified from
Sadowsky et al., 1976).

CONCLUSION

Finally, one important point remains to be discussed briefly—the relative
merits of clinical examination of the breast versus mammography. Two
clinical case histories will best illustrate this issue.

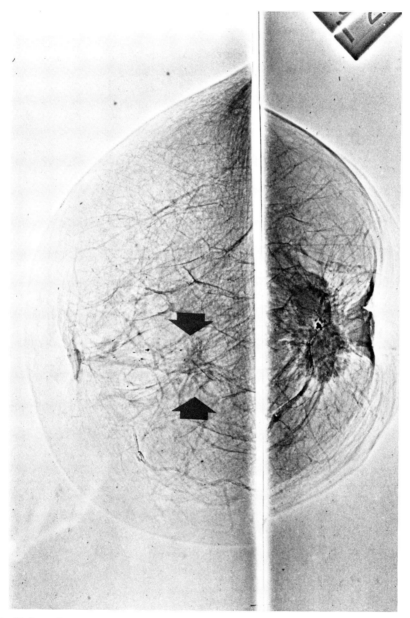

Fig. 23. Lateral mammograms of a patient with bilateral breast cancers. Note the obvious large tumor associated with nipple retraction in the right breast. The small scirrhous cancer in the left breast (arrows) was not apparent on physical examination.

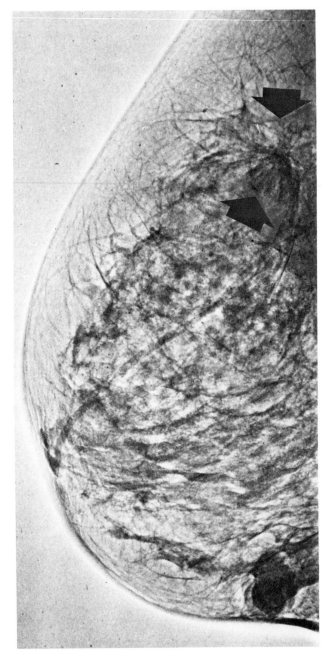

Fig. 24. Lateral mammogram showing a benign mass, a fibroadenoma, near the inferior skin fold of the breast. The second lesion, a small infiltrating cancer in the upper half of the breast (arrows), was not suspected clinically.

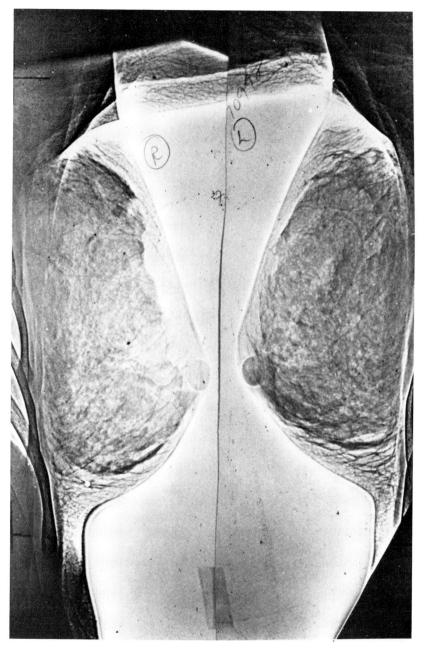

Fig. 25. Lateral mammograms of a young woman with severe breast dysplasia. A 3 cm cancer in the left breast is completely hidden by the density of the breast parenchyma.

Table II.
Indications for Mammography

1. The presence of a mass in a breast. As shown in Figures 23 and 24, a subclinical cancer can be found in the contra-lateral or ipsi-lateral breast.
2. A known diagnosis of cancer of one breast—i.e., post-mastectomy follow-up.
3. High-risk patient—family history of breast cancer, no children, mammary dysplasia, endometrial or ovarian cancer, early menarche, or late menopause.
4. Large, pendulous breasts that are difficult to examine clinically.
5. Other findings in the breast such as ulceration, dimpling, nipple discharge or retraction, and skin thickening.
6. Metastatic disease with an unknown primary tumor.
7. Cancerophobia.

The patient whose mammogram is shown in Figure 25 is a young woman with a clinically obvious discrete 3 cm mass in the left breast. The mammogram revealed dense breast parenchyma due to severe mammary dysplasia. In spite of several attempts and different views, no lesion could be demonstrated on the mammograms. The mass remained completely hidden by the dense breast tissue. There were no other helpful signs such as tumor calcifications or skin changes. The mass did prove to be a cancer on biopsy and a mastectomy was done.

An elderly asymptomatic woman had a screening mammogram (shown in Figure 26) done at the suggestion of her physician. On physical examination she had large pendulous breasts; otherwise the examination was completely unremarkable. The mammogram showed a small nodule, just under 1 cm in diameter, on the original film. This small nodule was found to be a mucinous carcinoma.

In general, it can be stated that the large fatty breast is the ideal subject for radiographic examination, which will yield the highest diagnostic accuracy, unlike physical examination which is difficult and unreliable on such a breast. The clinical examination, on the other hand, is much more reliable than a mammogram in a patient with small breasts or breasts with mammary dysplasia.

In summary, the two methods of breast examination, clinical palpation and mammography, are neither competitive nor exclusive of each other but *complementary.* Each method has its own limitations as well as its chief applications, which we must recognize and accept as such. Several published studies (Venet et al., 1969; Stark et al., 1974) address this problem. Their final conclusion is that the highest accuracy in breast cancer diagnosis will be obtained when both methods are properly used in the evaluation of the patient.

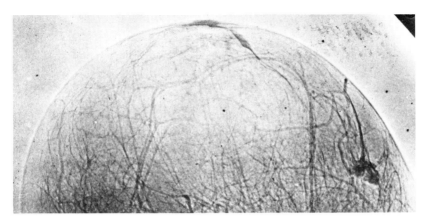

Fig. 26. Mammogram of a woman with large pendulous breasts. The small cancer, under 1 cm in diameter, was impossible to detect clinically but is seen clearly on the mammogram due to the fatty content of the breast.

REFERENCES

Egan, R. L. Fundamentals of mammographic diagnosis of benign and malignant diseases. *Oncology*. 23:126, 1969.

Egan, R. L. *Mammography*. Springfield, Ill.: Charles C. Thomas, 1964.

Egan, R. L. Experience with mammography in a tumor institution, evaluation of 1,000 studies. *Radiology*. 75:894, 1960.

Gershon-Cohen, J., Ingleby, H. *Comparative Anatomy, Pathology, and Roentgenology of the Breast*. Philadelphia: University of Pennsylvania Press, 1960.

Gershon-Cohen, J. and Ingelby, H. Carcinoma of the breast, roentgenographic technic and diagnostic criteria. *Radiology*. 60:68, 1953.

Gershon-Cohen, J. and Berger, S. M. Breast cancer with microcalcifications: diagnostic difficulties. *Radiology*. 87:613, 1966.

Golinger, R. C. Hormones and the pathophysiology of fibrocystic mastopathy. *Surgery, Gynecol., & Obstet*. 146:243, 1978.

Leborgne, R. Diagnosis of tumors of the breast by simple roentgenography. *Am. J. Roentgenol. & Rad. Therapy*. 65:1, 1951.

Rogers, J. V., Powell, W. R. Mammographic indications for biopsy of clinically normal breasts: correlation with pathologic findings in 72 cases. *Am. J. Roentgenol. & Rad. Therapy*. 115:794, 1972.

Sadowsky, N. L., Kalisher, L., White, G., Ferucci, J. T. Jr. Radiologic detection of breast cancer—review and recommendations. *New Eng. J. Med*. 294:370, 1976.

Stark, A. M., Way, S. The screening of well women for the detection of breast cancer using clinical examination with thermography and mammography. *Cancer*. 33:1671, 1974.

Venet, L., Strax, P., Venet, W., Shapiro, S. Adequacies and inadequacies of breast examinations by physicians. *Cancer*. 24:1187, 1969.

Wolfe, J. N. Breast patterns as an index of risk for developing breast cancer. *Am. J. Roentgenol. & Rad. Therapy*. 126:1130, 1976.

Wolfe, J. N. Xeroradiography of the breast. *Radiology*. 91:231, 1968.

Wolfe, J.N. *Mammography*. Springfield, Ill.: Charles C. Thomas, 1967.

CHAPTER 2

Risks Versus Benefits
Of Mammography

ABRAHAM GEFFEN

In 1963, the Health Insurance Plan of Greater New York (H.I.P.) initiated a study directed to the question "Does periodic breast cancer screening with mammographic and clinical examination result in a reduction in mortality from breast cancer in the female population?" (Shapiro et al., 1971, 1973). Two systematic random samples, each consisting of 31,000 women aged 40 to 64 years, were selected. Study group women were offered a screening examination and three additional annual examinations. Women in the control group followed their usual practices in receiving medical care.

Shapiro et al. (1973) reported that "over the short-run period of five years of follow-up, the study group of women have about a one-third lower mortality from breast cancer than those in the control group," and that "the screening program appears to have resulted in a reduction in breast cancer mortality in those at ages 50 and over but not at ages 40-49 years at the time of initial screening." These authors suggested the development of practical programs to screen for breast cancer as a high priority issue. In fact, the results of the H.I.P. study were considered a valid basis for extending breast cancer screening to a larger population under the sponsorship of the National Cancer Institute and the American Cancer Society. Twenty-seven Breast Cancer Detection Demonstration Projects (BCDDP) were started in 1973. These projects were to determine the experience in carrying out breast cancer screening in widely dispersed geographic areas of the U.S.

In January, 1976, Bailar (Bailar, 1976) raised serious questions concerning the relative risks versus benefits of including mammography in breast cancer screening. Bailar was concerned with certain biases which may diminish the reported beneficial effect of mammography in breast cancer screening—lead-time bias, length bias, and selectivity bias. Bailar presented the view that the improvement in mortality and survival rates as reported in the H.I.P. study, may be in actuality the result of lead-time bias and length bias.

Lead-time is the amount of time by which diagnosis is advanced by screening. Lead-time may vary among subgroups detected on screening. A completely satisfactory technique for adjusting for lead-time bias is not presently known.

Length bias results from the fact that with screening there is a high probability of detecting cases with relatively long preclinical durations. Bailar (1976) indicated that breast cancer cases detected on screening are more likely than others to have long preclinical durations. Such patients who have been screened will tend to have tumors that progress slowly and will tend to live longer than others. Bailar indicated that these neoplasms will tend to have other characteristics of a good prognosis, such as below-average involvement of regional lymph nodes and a relatively high degree of differentiation. He added that "it must be understood that these are inherent characteristics of the disease that increase the likelihood of cancer being detected at screening, rather than beneficial effects of screening resulting from detection at an earlier time."

Selectivity bias results if self-selection for screening is allowed without a suitable control study group, as exemplified in the HIP study.

Bailar was also concerned with the risk of cancer induction due to radiation carcinogenesis, citing for evidence the epidemiological studies which will be outlined below in detail. He reemphasized the evaluations of the United Nations Scientific Committee on the Effects of Atomic Radiation (UNSCEAR) 1972 and of the National Academy of Sciences-National Research Council Committee on the Biological Effects of Ionizing Radiation (BEIR, 1972) pertaining to mammography. Bailar's effective espousal of the risks over the benefits of x-ray mammography for screening, even prior to his published article, was a prime stimulus for the wave of stories in the press and television that led to the refusal of many women to undergo mammography when recommended for diagnostic reasons. The media's impact was even greater in discouraging women from having mammography for screening.

Even prior to the publication of Bailar's article, in response to the questions concerning risks versus benefits of mammography for screening of patients for breast cancer, in 1975 Dr. Guy R. Newell, M.D., deputy director of the National Cancer Institute, appointed three distinguished scientists to direct three Working Groups on Mammography Screening for Breast Cancer as follows:

To direct the epidemiology and biostatistics group, he appointed Lester Breslow, M.D., to be Chairman. Breslow is dean of the School of Public Health, University of California in Los Angeles. Named chairman of the pathology group was Louis B. Thomas, M.D., chief of the Laboratory of Pathology, National Cancer Institute, Bethesda, Md. And the appointed chairman of the radiation and carcinogenesis group was Arthur C. Upton, M.D., director of the National Cancer Institute.

The following is a summary of their final report: (Breslow et al., 1977):

REVIEW OF EVIDENCE FOR RISKS

There is evidence for a radiation-induced excess of breast cancer in women who have had irradiation, based on epidemiological studies in the following:

a) women who received multiple fluoroscopic examinations of the chest in the treatment of pulmonary tuberculosis with artificial pneumothorax;

b) women given x-ray therapy to the breast for postpartem mastitis; and

c) Japanese women exposed to atomic-bomb irradiation.

1) Studies in Nova Scotia (Myrden et al., 1969; Myrden et al., 1974) have revealed 36 breast cancers in 308 women who had fluoroscopy and were followed for up to 32 years after initial exposure, as compared with eight cancers in a control group of 493 women who did not have fluoroscopy and who were followed for a comparable period. The quantitative estimate of the risk (11th to 28th year, since no cancers appeared before ten years) corresponds to 8.5 cases of breast cancer per 1 million person years per rad (BEIR Report, 1972).

These observations have been confirmed by two other series, one in Ontario (Cook et al., 1974) and one in Massachusetts (Boice et al., 1978). In the latter study, in 1047 women who had fluoroscopy during pneumothorax treatment for pulmonary tuberculosis between 1930 and 1954, the incidence of breast cancer was higher (41 cases observed, versus 23.3 expected on the basis of rates derived from the Connecticutt tumor registry) than that in a comparison group of 717 women who did not have fluoroscopy (15 cases observed versus 14.1 expected). For 10 to 44 years after radiation exposure, the overall risk was estimated at 6.2 cases per million person years per rad. The authors also concluded that when breast cancer risk is considered as a function of absorbed dose in the breast, instead of as a function of the number of fluoroscopic examinations, a linear dose-response relationship over the range of estimated dose is consistent with the data.

There is one series (Delarue et al., 1975) that shows no excess of breast cancer in a group of Canadian women subjected to multiple fluoroscopies. The number in this series, however, is so small that the results are not as significant as those in the three series already cited.

2) Mettler et al., (1969) first reported on the increase of cancer of the breast in women who had been treated with x-rays for postpartum mastitis. This work has been extended to include three groups of non-irradiated con-

trols (Shore et al., 1976). In the 571 women who had irradiation the risk was estimated at 8.3 cases per million person years per rad. This figure is similar to the estimate derived from the Nova Scotia study and higher than that in the Massachusetts report, cited above, on women developing cancer of the breast following multiple fluoroscopic examinations of the chest in the treatment of pulmonary tuberculosis with artificial pneumothorax.

3) The studies of Japanese women exposed to atomic-bomb irradiation (Wanebo et al., 1968; McGregor et al., 1977) revealed 187 cases of breast cancer, corresponding to 2.4 cases per million person years per rad. The value for the Japanese women is lower than the value for the North American women (series cited above), possibly for reasons associated with the much lower natural incidence of breast cancer in Japanese women.

In an analysis of the above evidence, the Breslow-Thomas-Upton report (1977) discussed the dose-response relationship, reviewing experimental animal radiation-induced mammary carcinogenesis. The authors concluded that there are no radiobiologic grounds for postulating the existence of a threshold dose for carcinogenesis and that linear dose response-curves are valid (Rossi et al., 1972). The evidence derived from the human data referred to above also supports a linear dose-response curve (Bailar, 1977; Boice et al., 1978; McGregor et al., 1977).

The Report (1977) further concludes that based on the evidence cited and the assumption that the dose-response remains linear irrespective of dose, dose rate, and age at irradiation, along with an adjustment for the effects of age differences in susceptibility, "the risk of mammography may be assumed to approximate 3.5 to 7.5 cases of breast cancer per million women of age 35 or older at risk per year per rad to both breasts from the tenth year after irradiation throughout the remainder of life" (Breslow, Thomas, Upton Report 1977, page 36).

Expressed from the viewpoint of the individual, a single mammography performed using the low-dose technique (administering average dose to the breast of less than one rad) would increase the lifetime probability of developing cancer from an average risk of 7.58% to a level of about 7.59% to 7.61% or by 1% at age 35 and by a progressively smaller percentage with increasing age at examination thereafter (idem). This value is based on one rad dose or less per examination, and applies only to the better-than-average exposure situation today.

REVIEW OF BENEFITS OF MAMMOGRAPHY IN SCREENING

The Breslow-Thomas-Upton groups (1977) evaluated the H.I.P. of Greater New York cancer screening project to determine the gross and net benefits of adding mammography to history-taking and physical examinations. Shapiro (1977) in his report on seven-year mortality data from the HIP study, showed a reduction of 46% in women aged 50 to 59 years, almost identical to the mortality rate for women aged 40 to 49 years. Clinical examination and mammography contributed independently; 33% of the breast cancers would have been missed if mammography had not been included, and 45% of all cases detected at screening would have been missed without clinical examination. A reasonable estimate of the independent contribution of mammography is a 10% to 15% reduction in breast cancer mortality for women over age 50 (Shapiro et al., 1971, 1973).

The net benefit, based on risks (six cases per 1 million women per year per rad after a ten-year latent period) and 15% benefit over age 50, is progressively significant from age 50 and up, but definitely a negative benefit for women between the ages of 35 and 50 (Breslow, Thomas, Upton Groups Reports, 1977).

Based on these conclusions, the Breslow-Thomas-Upton working groups recommended discontinuing routine screening of women under the age of 50. Their recommendations in turn had immediate and serious effects. The Division of Cancer Control and Rehabilitation of the National Cancer Institute established a new working group to conduct an extensive review of the National Cancer Institute-American Cancer Society Breast Cancer Detection Demonstration Projects (BCDDP) on the basis of data accumulated from the 29 projects.

SUMMARY OF REPORT OF WORKING GROUP TO REVIEW THE NCI/ACS BCDDP

The new working group (known as the BCDDP Review Group) was formed on January 31, 1977, with Dr. Oliver H. Baehrs, M.D., consultant in surgery at the Mayo Clinic and professor of surgery at the Mayo Medical School, as chairman. Two sub-groups were organized. Named chairman of the epidemiology and statistics group was Sam Shapiro, director of the health services research and development center at the Johns Hopkins Medical Institution and professor of the health services administration, School of Hygiene and Public Health.

Charles Smart, M.D., chief of surgery at the Latter-Day Saints Hospital, Salt Lake City, Utah, was appointed chairman of the clinical review group. The results of these groups were published September 6, 1977 (Baehrs Report 1977). Some of the significant results are listed:
· 261,859 women had been screened as of June 30, 1976.
· 966 breast cancers were detected.

• 43.9% of the breast cancers were detected by mammography alone.
• 7.4% of the breast cancers were detected by physical examination only.
• One-third of the cancers were minimal (less than 1 cm in diameter).
• 60% of the minimal cancers were detected by mammography only.
• 70% of the minimal cancers had negative lymph nodes.
• One-third of the cancers were in the below-50 age group.
• 40% of the below-50 age group cancers were detected by mammography only.

The BCDDP review group concluded that mammography and physical examination combined is an effective procedure in detecting early breast cancer among women under 50 as well as among those over 50.

As the various BCDDP groups tabulate and report their results, more light may be shed on this dilemma of risks versus benefits of mammography for breast cancer screening. Fox et al., (1978) have written an incisive critique based on data from the Cincinnati and Milwaukee BCDDP Projects. They feel that the HIP study is not indicative of what mammography can offer young women because of improvements in technique since the study. On the other hand, BCDDP results are limited because significant mortality data are not yet available. A serious criticism of the BCDDP is the lack of a control study group. This pertains to three major problems:

1) The clinical incidence rate for the screened population is not known. (There may be self-selection of high risk groups and regional biases.)

2) The number of symptomatic women is not known.

3) There is no easily available reference group with which to compare survival data.

Fox et al. (1978) calculate a mathematical benefit/risk ratio for five annual mammographic examinations in women aged 35 to 49. Their estimates are: "worst case" 3.4 ± 1.1/1; "most probable" 8.0 ± 3.1/1. This is an attempt to quantitate the benefit/risk ratio (the benefit varying from two to 11 times the risk) depending on certain variable but known factors.

RECOMMENDATIONS OF CONSENSUS PANEL

Following receipt of the reports of all of the working groups (Breslow-Thomas-Upton and BCDDP review groups), the National Cancer Institute of the National Institutes of Health conducted a 16-member consensus development panel to examine the issues and the state of the art of breast cancer screening. The panel, which met on September 14-16, 1977, in Bethesda, Md., consisted of clinicians, scientists, and lay people. The chairman was Samuel O. Thier, M.D., professor and chairman of the department of internal medicine, Yale University. The panel reviewed the National Cancer Institute ad hoc working group reports and the BCDDP working group reports and heard many presentations and discussions. (Thier, 1977)

Acknowledging that mammography has improved markedly in recent years with marked reduction in radiation dose, the panel accepted the report of Dr. A.C. Upton, then head of the ad hoc working group studying the risk of radiation exposure. That report stated that current evidence strongly suggests a direct linear relationship between the amount of radiation and the risk of developing cancer, placing a presumptive risk from exposure to the breast at less than 1% per rad. This implies that a mammogram using the current low-dose technique would increase a woman's lifetime risk of breast cancer from an average natural level of about 7% to a level of less than 7.07%.

The consensus panel (Statement, 1977) made the following recommendations:

1) Continue BCDDP routine annual screening of women 50 years of age and older.

2) Women 40 to 49 years of age should be offered mammography in screening only if they have prior histories of breast cancer or if their mother or sister(s) have such histories.

3) Mammography for women 35 to 39 years of age should be restricted to those with histories of breast cancer.

4) The value of mammography as used in diagnosis for evaluating symptoms of clinical signs of breast cancer, such as the presence of a lump, swelling, discharge, dimpling, thickening, or other abnormality in the breast, has not been questioned.

CONCLUSION

What can be concluded from this review of the findings of the prestigious panelists who have studied the dilemma of risks versus benefits in the use of mammography for screening? Even though there may be some unanswered questions, a pragmatic approach is suggested. Guidance is available to the clinician whose advice is sought by the patient with concerns about breast cancer.

For diagnostic purposes, to evaluate symptoms or clinical signs of breast cancer, mammography should not be avoided.

For screening patients over the age of 50, mammography is advisable. For screening patients under age 50, if the patient is from 40 to 49 years old, mammography should be advised if there is a prior history of breast cancer or if the patient's mother or sister(s) have such a history; if the patient is from 35 to 39 years old, mammography should be advised only if she herself has a history of breast cancer.

These recommendations represent a consensus, based on present knowledge. These guidelines may change with time and with accumulation of more knowledge.

REFERENCES

Baehrs, O. H., Shapiro, S., and Smart, C. Report of the Working Group to Review the NCI/ACS Breast Cancer Detection Demonstration Projects. Sept. 6, 1977

Bailar, J.C., III. Mammography: a contrary view. *Ann. Int. Med.* 84:77, 1976.

Bailar, J. C., III. Screening for early breast cancer: pros and cons (in Proceedings of the Conference on Breast Cancer: A Report to the profession.) *Cancer* 39 (6) Supplement: 2783, 1977.

BEIR Report. Report of the advisory committee on the biological effects of ionizing radiations: The effects on populations of exposures to low levels of ionizing radiation. Wash., D.C. Division of Medical Sciences, National Academy of Sciences, National Ressearch Council, Nov. 1972.

Boice, J.D. Jr., Rosenstein, M., Trout, E.D. Estimation of breast doses and breast cancer risk associated with repeated fluoroscopic chest examinations of women with tuberculosis. *Radiat. Res.* 73:373, 1978.

Breslow, L., Thomas, L.B., Upton, A.C. Reports of National Cancer Institute Ad Hoc Committee Working Groups on Mammography Screening for Breast Cancer. U.S. Dept. of H.E.W. Publication No. (NIH) 77-1400. March, 1977.

Cook, D.C., Dent, C., Hewitt, D. Breast cancer following multiple chest fluoroscopy: the Ontario experience. *Can. Med. Assoc. J.* 111:406, 1974.

Delarue, N.C., Gale, G., Ronald, A. Multiple fluoroscopy of the chest: carcinogenicity for the female breast and implications for breast cancer screening programs. *Can. Med. Assoc. J.* 112:1405, 1975.

Fox, S.H., Moskowitz, M., Saenger, E.L., Kereiakes, J.G., Milbrath, J., and Goodwin, M.W. Benefit/Risk analysis of aggressive mammographic screening. *Radiology* 128:359, 1978.

McGregor, D.H., Land, C.E., Tokuoqa, S., Liu, P., Wakabayashi, T., Beebe, G.W. Breast cancer incidence among atomic bomb survivors, Hiroshima and Nagasaki, 1950-1969 J. Nat. Canc. Inst. 59:799, 1977

Mettler, F.A., Hempelmann, L.H., Dutton, A.M., Pifer, J.W., Toyooka, E.T., Ames, W.R. Breast neoplasms in women treated with x-rays for acute postpartum mastitis. A pilot study. *J. Nat. Canc. Inst.* 43:803, 1969.

Myrden, J.A. and Quinlan, J.J. Breast carcinoma following multiple fluoroscopies with pneumothorax treatment of pulmonary tuberculosis. *Ann. R. Coll. Phys. Can.* 7:45, 1974.

Myrden, J.A., Hiltz, J.E. Breast cancer following multiple fluoroscopies during artificial pneumothorax treatment of pulmonary tuberculosis. *Can. Med. Assoc. J.* 100:1032, 1969.

Rossi, H.H. Kellerer, A.M. Radiation carcinogenesis at low doses, *Science* 175:200, 1972.

Shapiro, S., Strax, P., and Venet, L. Periodic breast cancer screening in reducing mortality from breast cancer. *J.A.M.A.* 215:1777, 1971.

Shapiro, S., Strax, P., Venet, L., Venet, W. Changes in five-year breast cancer mortality in a breast cancer screening program. In Seventh National Cancer Conference Proceedings, Philadelphia: J.B. Lippincott, 1973, pp. 673-678.

Shapiro, S. In Breslow, Thomas, Upton Report of Working Groups on Mammography in Screening for Breast Cancer. U.S. D. of H.E.W. Publication No. (NIH) 77-1400. pp. 3-5. March, 1977.

Shore, R.E., Hempelmann, L.H., Kowaluk, E., Mansur, P.S., Pasternack, B.S., Albert, R.E., Haughie, G.E. Breast neoplasms in women treated with x-rays for acute postpartum mastitis. J. Nat. Canc. Inst. 59:813, 1977.

Thier, S. Report (Statement) of Consensus Development Panel on Breast Cancer Screening. U.S. Dept. of H.E.W., National Cancer Institute, National Institutes of Health, Oct. 15, 1977.

UNSCEAR - United Nations Scientific Committee on the Effects of Atomic Radiation. Ionizing Radiation: Levels and Effects. Vol. 2: Effects. N.Y., United Nations, 1972.

Wanebo, C.K., Johnson, K.C., Sato, K., Thorshud, T.W. Breast cancer after exposure to the atomic bombings of Hiroshima and Nagasaki. *New Eng. J. Med.* 279:667, 1968.

CHAPTER 3

Mass Screening In Control Of Breast Cancer

PHILIP STRAX

RATIONALE

The ideal method for control of breast cancer is primary prevention. If we knew the initiating cause of the disease, we might be able to prevent its development. No such information is on the horizon. Another approach could be total eradication of breast cancer regardless of the stage at detection. This possibility also eludes us. All we have is the common knowledge that detection of the disease at a localized stage, when there is no clinical evidence of nodal or other organ involvement, leads to at least an 85% survival rate at five years. When the disease is not localized the 5-year survival rate drops to 50% or less.

It is also generally believed that breast cancer exists in a prepalpable stage for a varying period of time. Detection of the disease before it can be felt by the woman or her physician carries with it a particularly good prognosis. In a practical way, finding breast cancer before it becomes palpable requires screening of apparently healthy women. That is the rationale of the mass screening programs being conducted today.

The impetus for this approach has been the results of the Health Insurance Plan H.I.P. of Greater New York study which has indicated a persistent one-third reduction of mortality in a study group compared to a matched control group. This program demonstrated the value of mass screening as a method for saving lives of women from breast cancer by detecting the disease at an early stage.

PROBLEM

Breast cancer now represents 28% of all malignancies in women, making it the most common cancer of any bodily part. Today one in every 13 women develops the disease. Thirty years ago the figure was one in 20. Breast cancer has been increasing in incidence by 1% a year for the past 10 years. It is still the number one cause of death in women aged 39 to 44. It remains the number one cancer killer of women at any age. It increases in incidence with age. What is even more important is that regardless of advances in diagnosis and treatment, there has been a persistent stationary death rate from the disease in the past 40 years, although during this period deaths from all causes in women have been declining.

An important reason for this poor showing may be that over 90% of breast cancer is first detected by the women themselves, who bring the problem to their physicians after a more or less delayed period. It seems obvious that since most breast cancer today is not localized when first seen by the clinician, a means must be found to have women present themselves for examination when the disease is at an earlier stage then is commonly the case. This means, in a practical way, detection of preclinical cancer in apparently "well" women, when the disease is unsuspected by patient or physician—as is true in mass screening.

REMEDY

Screening as defined by the World Health Organization, is "the presumptive identification of unrecognized disease or defect by the application of tests, examination or other procedures which can be applied rapidly. Screening tests sort our apparently well persons who probably have a disease from those who probably do not. A screening test is not intended to be diagnostic. Persons with positive or suspicious findings must be referred to their physicians for diagnosis and necessary treatment." It should be noted that by definition, unrecognized symptomatic, as well as presymptomatic disease, is included. Tests may be diagnostic, though not necessarily so intended. Thus, mammography or palpation is covered by this definition, provided it is rapidly carried out.

From the 1940s through the 1960s studies by many investigators (Day et al., 1961; Gilbertson et al., 1971; Holleb et al., 1960) concluded that periodic mass screening for breast cancer led to improved survival statistics. Only inspection and palpation were involved at that time because mammography was not in common usage. These studies included 30% of "interval" cancers found within a year of an apparently negative examination. Today we suspect that most of these could have been found as nonpalpable cancers on mammography.

In the early 1960s Gershon-Cohen, et al. (1961) as well as others (Friedman et al., 1966; Stevens et al., 1966) discussed the use of mammography as a screening procedure in breast cancer with mixed results. All reported detecting occult, nonpalpable cancer, especially on periodic study. Their conclusions varied from enthusiastic acceptance to mild approval of the procedure for women over the age of 50. Most felt that the cost and effort of mass screening was too great for the resultant benefit.

These studies suffered from a lack of a combined approach using both clinical examination and mammography and from an absence of a control group for true evaluation of the potential of mass screening in mortality reduction. Only a definitive study, such as the H.I.P. investigation involving large enough numbers of women and containing a built-in matched control group, could provide the data needed to conclude that mass screening might save lives.

In the study conducted by the H.I.P. under contract with the National Cancer Institute, there has been a persistent one-third reduction in mortality in a study group of 31,000 randomly selected women from a registry of women aged 40 to 64, as compared to a matched control group (Shapiro et al., 1973).

In a nine year follow-up of breast cancer found within five years of diagnosis, 128 deaths from breast cancer occurred in the control group compared with 91 in the study group women, only two-thirds of whom actually responded to the invitation for examination. These data formed the basis for expanding the concept of mass screening for detection of early and more localized breast cancer as a means for saving lives of women from this disease.

All those examined in the H.I.P. study received independent mammography and clinical examination. The importance of mammography was emphasized by the fact that of 44 cancers found only on the x-ray, only three women have died of breast cancer in a nine-year follow-up. Of all the cancers detected through screening in this study one third were found on mammography alone and were not felt by palpation. However, it should also be emphasized that two-fifths of the cancers were found on clinical examination alone and were not detected by the x-ray. Obviously, both modalities were necessary for proper yield. It is also important to note that the cancers found on one modality alone had a high percentage of no axillary nodal involvement — 79% in those found on mammography alone and 75% in those detected by clinical examination alone. It appears that in early breast cancer only one modality may be positive in a high percentage of cases. Cancers found on both modalities had the same percentage of positive nodes (over 50%) as in the control group.

Another important finding was that 15% of the cancers found in the study developed within 12 months after an apparently negative examination.

These so-called "interval" cancers had the same rate of nodal involvement as the control group. In subsequent screening programs, this factor needed further attention.

It was particularly noteworthy that the entire reduction in mortality was concentrated in women over the age of 50. Those women under 50 showed no such improvement. Mammography is less effective in younger women when the breasts are more glandular and more dense on the mammograms.

These facts pointed to three areas of potential improvement in considering further mass screening efforts in the general population:

1) Emphasis needed to be placed on breast self-examination. It was this procedure that could detect the "interval" cancer in an earlier stage. The woman herself needed to become our ally in detection of breast cancer. It was felt strongly that this procedure needed to be taught to women directly on a one-to-one basis. The pamphelets distributed over the years by the cancer societies were just not enough.

2) Improvement in mammography was needed particularly to produce greater resolution and contrast in mammograms of young women and with reduced radiation.

3) The thermogram, as introduced by Lawson (1956) of Montreal, was an additional modality that could alert the clinician to the possibility of abnormality in one breast as compared with the other. Its addition as another detection modality needed evaluation.

These considerations led to the development in 1968 of the Guttman Breast Diagnostic Institute in New York City with the basic objective of developing a mass screening approach that would be feasible and could reach the general population of women. The two major problems to be solved were: how to develop a practical, economical, and efficient method that could produce satisfactory yield of early cancers and how to motivate women to accept such a procedure.

A tandem approach (Strax, 1975; Strax, 1976; Strax, 1977) has been developed: an interview (for data on demography, health, breast and menstrual history), a clinical examination, mammography, and thermography. Breast self-examination, is taught to women being screened directly on a one-to-one basis at the time of palpation.

Those with questionable findings (not sufficiently suspicious to warrant intervention) are recalled in three to six months. All data are sent to a physician chosen by the woman. Follow-up is emphasized. All biopsy recommendations are carefully followed for surgical results. Those women not having biopsies are recalled in three months.

Examinations are conducted on New York City women with the cooperation of the American Cancer Society (New York City Division), which has been most helpful in stimulating motivation.

The three methods used in screening for breast cancer are clinical examination, including palpation and inspection, mammography, and thermography.

Clinical Examination

Clinical examination is an essential feature in screening for breast cancer. However, with palpation it is particularly difficult to locate the presumably early and small cancers, which often have characteristics associated with a benign lesion. The clinician must be aware of this potential pitfall, which is particularly great in the postmenopausal woman with large breasts.

A substantial number of cancers that are palpable are not detectable with our present mammographic techniques. Therefore, if a clinical examination indicates a possible lesion, a negative mammogram must never deter the clinician from exploration. The value of palpation in screening is in direct proportion to the expertise of the examiner. All physicians involved in screening should assiduously cultivate the art of clinical examination, which may be the sole indicator of cancer in a curable stage. (Venet et al., 1971)

Mammography

The female breast is readily accessible to inspection and palpation. Why then do we need mammography? (Strax, 1975).

1) The breast is normally a multi-nodular structure, which practically always is made up of varying-sized small or large "lumps." The dominant mass that suggests pathology may not be clearly evident on inspection or palpation. This is particularly true of an early cancer. The mammogram is our most useful modality that very often—not always—gives the physician that extra assurance that he may be dealing with a malignant (or benign) process. It is often the added bit of suspicion that leads to prompt exploration.

2) In the face of a clinically definite lesion that is about to be explored, the mammogram can yield additional information about the rest of the breast or about the opposite breast. There may be lurking elsewhere in either breast a cancer which is completely nonpalpable, and this other lesion may be the cancer, not the mass leading to exploration.

3) One of the most cogent reasons for mammography, particularly in the symptomatic woman who feels a vague mass, severe localized pain, or nipple discharge, is the varied expertise of physicians in the clinical examination of breasts.

4) It has been known for many years that a breast cancer may not be palpable by even the most expert hands and yet be in the early stages of a deadly disease. The breast cancer screening activities, mammography in addition to clinical examination, that have been going on for about 15 years, have turned up hundreds of such lesions. It is these nonpalpable cancers, which have a high degree of no nodal involvement and are accompanied by a substantially increased survival rate and often a reduced mortality rate, that have brought the importance of the x-ray examination of the breast to the fore.

Xeromammography (Wolfe, 1972) is merely a variation of mammography in which the same x-rays are used to produce the image. A charged selenium plate is used instead of film and the end result is a mammographic image on paper with considerable edge-enhancement. There is a difference of opinion among radiologists about the superiority of the two display mediums, some preferring one and some the other. Most experienced mammographers think the micro-calcifications may be more easily detected on the xerox plate but that masses are more easily detected on the improved film of mammography.

Thermography

Thermography is a useful modality in breast cancer diagnosis in a more peripheral manner. It detects physiological changes resulting in increased heat which is measured by special heat sensors and translated into a photographic image. Many breast conditions (both benign and malignant) are associated with increased heat. Thermography is thus not an indicator of cancer as such. It does alert the clinician to the possibility of the disease. The increased heat areas do not necessarily correspond to the location of the cancer, however, and thus exploration cannot be performed on the basis of an abnormal thermogram alone. Clinical examination or mammography is needed for more definite diagnosis and localization.

Thermography can be of great help, however, in the case that is otherwise doubtful. A hot thermogram will tend to encourage exploration and thus avoid missing an early case. Some 20% to 25% of abnormal thermograms are found in patients with no abnormal findings on the other modalities. These women need to be watched more closely and may represent a high-risk group. Some observers have found occasional cancers becoming apparent clinically one to two years after positive thermography results (Fink et al., 1978; Isard et al., 1974; Moskowitz et al., 1976).

In the diagnosis of breast cancer, thermography should never be used alone, even as a prescreening method. It is particularly ineffective in detecting the very early nonpalpable cancer. It may be of value as an ancillary method for detection of breast abnormalities particularly in a tandem approach with clinical examination and mammography.

A recent joint statement by the American College of Radiology and the American Thermographic Society defines thermography as a "complementary diagnostic tool that may be useful in evaluation of breast disease when combined with both physical examination under the supervision of a qualified physician and mammography by a trained radiologist.

Ultrasound

The use of ultrasound is still in the exploratory stage. The method may be developed to the point where it could be useful to add to the program or replace modalities now being used.

Radiation Dosage

In recent years there has been a dramatic improvement both in the quality of mammography and in the radiation dose used. The most widely used technique, purporting to produce the highest quality, in the 1960s was that of Egan (1962). The procedure involved a slow industrial Kodak type M film, a tungsten tube, close coning, no compression with low kilvoltage and high milliampere-seconds. This technique produced high quality mammograms with radiation doses ranging from 7 to 12 rads to the skin per examination. In the last few years, under the leadership of British radiologists, including Price et al. (1975) and Ostrum et al. (1973) among others in the U.S., the use of faster film-screen combinations in vacuum cassettes has seen a remarkable improvement in contrast and in resolution of the mammographic image plus a reduction in radiation to levels of 0.2 to 0.3 rad to the skin.

The latest measurements by Miller and associates (Miller et al., 1977) indicate that such skin radiation, with the low kilovoltages used plus the molybdenum-anode tubes and compression techniques, is delivering doses to the mid breast of .02 to .03 rads for a right angle pair of fims. These techniques are readily available and are being used by an increasing number of radiologists. Revision of techniques in xeromammography, with the introduction of the negative node and increase of kilovoltage, has resulted in reduction of radiation, although not to the low levels attainable by the newer film-screen techniques.

Wilkinson and associates (1978) using Xerg (Xonics) techniques, have produced high quality mammograms with radiation markedly reduced to levels even lower than those of the best of the film-screen techniques. This process holds great promise for the development of mammography techniques with radiation dosages so low as to be negligible in comparison with the potential benefit of the x-ray study of the breast.

Radiation Hazard

Attention was called by Bailar (1976) to the potential radiation hazard of mammography. However, the recent innuendoes and unwarranted statements concerning the radiation hazard of mammography are developing a new danger—the danger of *not* doing mammography when necessary. Thousands of women of all ages—over 50 as well as under 50—with signs and symptoms of disease as well as those without disease have been refusing mammography and even palpation as a result of the hysteria engendered by the mammography controversy. There is already evidence that cancers have been detected at a later stage than they could have been had women not been frightened away. In considering the controversy, the following factors should be borne in mind:

It is generally agreed that:

1) The symptomatic woman with a dominant mass, localized pain, or nipple discharge always has the real possibility of harboring a cancer. All diagnostic means, including mammography, must be used for elucidation of the problem.

2) Since the H.I.P. study demonstrated a substantial reduction in mortality in women over the age of 50 (40% in this group), the great value of mammography as part of a periodic screening program in this age group has been widely recognized. Particularly when considering the use of the newer low-dosage mammography techniques, it has been widely accepted that mammography is proper and necessary as part of a routine health examination in all women over the age of 50.

The only group about which there is real disagreement on whether mammography is ethically indicated is the one containing women aged under 50 who are truly asymptomatic. However, there is general agreement that when such women have the substantial risk factors of previous breast cancer or a positive family history in a mother or sister, they should have periodic complete examinations, including mammography. Of course, since breast cancer is uncommon in women under the age of 35, they should be excluded unless medical suspicion of breast disease warrants mammography.

The problem in the young asymptomatic woman revolves about two facts:

1) The breast is sensitive to irradiation. Previous studies on women subjected to substantial doses of radiation, such as from the atomic bomb, from fluoroscopy in the course of tuberculosis treatment, or from radiation treatment for breast abscess, have indicated an increased incidence of the disease in women exposed. Such breast cancer initiation had a latent period of about 10 years and varied in proportion to dose.

Although no evidence exists for the absence of a threshold dose, it has been considered prudent that such a dose be postulated and that a linear radiation effect be asssumed down to the smallest quantity of radiation. It has been stated that "1 rad to the body of the breast given to a million women would produce six cancers per year for a lifetime of the woman after a latent period of six to 10 years" by Dr. Arthur Upton, noted radiobiologist and director of the National Cancer Institute. This seems a fair statement of radiation risk from mammography.

2) There has been no evidence to date that the H.I.P. study, using clinical examination and mammography with the techniques considered optimum at the time, has produced any reduction in mortality from breast cancer in women under age 50. Whether such a state of affairs would exist in the National Cancer Institute-American Cancer Society screening programs with the improved mammographic techniques being used must be considered pure supposition.

In considering risks versus benefits in mammography, emphasis should be placed on four additional factors:

1. Radiation Risk

Risk is directly proportional to dose. The state of the art of mammography has changed radically in the years since the H.I.P. study. In that study doses of 8 R to the skin were given per examination. New filmscreen techniques, as used at the Guttman Institute and elsewhere, now deliver 0.2 to 0.3 R to the skin per exposure or, as we have noted above, doses of about .02 to .03 rads to the mid breast for two views.

Using .02 to .03 rad for a complete examination of the breast, instead of 1 rad in the formula mentioned above means that if all 40 million women at risk for breast cancer in the U.S. were to receive a breast examination, including mammography, every year for up to 30 years, as would be the case for the youngest women being exposed, the following would happen: The usual present incidence of 90,000 breast cancers and 34,000 deaths from the disease would be found. With screening (using mammography plus palpation) we would reduce the death rate by at least one-third, or save 12,000 lives. The cost from the radiation would be six patients per year, or 180 patients in the 30 years of lifetime, after a 10-year latent period. And one-third of these would probably be saved. In other words, *at least* 12,000 women would be salvaged at a cost of, *at most,* 120 lives over 30 years. In short, such a dosage is negligible by all radiologic standards and should permit more liberal interpretation of risks versus benefits.

2. Mammography Benefit

The absence of a statistical mortality benefit in women under age 50 is an important factor in the guidelines limiting mammography in this age group. Let us consider this further:

In the H.I.P. study more cancers were found in the study group than in the control group in women under age 50 when comparing age of diagnosis. Yet the numbers of cancers at age of death were the same. Perhaps in women under 50, cancers of the more localized type, found particularly on mammography in the study group, might have been detected over the age of 50 at a more advanced stage if no screening program had been available.

Perhaps screening women under age 50 in that study helped to keep the death rate down in those women over 50. This concept is being investigated further. It may elucidate the perplexing question of why mortality benefit was demonstrated only in women over 50 years of age.

3. Symptomatic Women

The guidelines specifically exclude women with any symptoms "whatsoever." This gray area needs further clarification. When does a lump or a pain or a nipple discharge make a woman symptomatic? Is a single lump a symptom and lumpiness or multiple lumps not? Is a localized persistent pain a symptom and diffuse intermittent pai not? Is a free-flowing dark discharge a symptom and a discharge produced by nipple pressure not? Is a "symptomatic" woman the one who goes to a physician for a breast examination and not the one who goes to a breast center like the Guttman Institute? These are important considerations, certainly in the mind of the woman. Minor degrees of symptoms are commonplace. When we consider that most cancers are found under screening auspices in women under age 50 as well as in women over age 50 with only minimal symptoms or none at all, can we not begin to be more liberal with our interpretation in light of the low breast radiation dose?

4. Other Risk Factors

Women in general are at varying risk of developing breast cancer. Age, of course, is a most important factor. The value of mammography as a detector of breast cancer increases with age. There is very little breast cancer in women under age 35. After that, the risk for breast cancer development increases with age. Other risk factors of varying strength include:

a) Presence of a dominant lump, localized pain, or nipple discharge. Many authorities include "chronic mastitis" with or without pain (Copeland, 1978).
b) History of previous breast cancer.
c) Positive family history—especially of premenopausal breast cancer.
d) No children or birth of a first child after the age of 30.
e) Early menarche (before age 11) or late menopause.
f) Less well-known factors such as being Jewish, of European extraction, in the middle- or upper-income bracket, or postmenopausally obese.

It should be emphasized that in any large series of breast cancers, especially those detected under screening auspices, the majority of malignancies are found in women who have none of the risk factors listed above, with the exception, perhaps, of minor symptoms. However, the presence of any of the above factors increases the need for periodic surveillance.

RESULTS

Guttman Institute

Of 162,876 examinations made from 1971 to 1976, 70,467 were initial studies and 92,409 were subsequent examinations. Of 5,534 recommendations for biopsy or aspiration, 3,624 were done and 846 cancers were found.

On initial examination, the proportion of prevalent cancers present was high (8.4 cancers per 1,000), depending on such factors as self-selection and age of women. Because cancers had been present for varying lengths of time, only 48% of the cancers were free of nodal involvement. On subsequent examination, the proportion of incident cancers, which had become detectable after the previous exam, was 2.7 per 1,000, but 74% had no nodal spread (Table I).

Use of the tandem technique (clinical examination supplemented by mammography and thermography) showed that 20% of the cancers were found by mammography alone, 22% by clinical examination alone, and 58% by both (Table II). As in the H.I.P. study, 70% of women with cancers

Table I.
Value of Periodic Examinations

Number of Examinations (1971-1976)				162,876		

Age distribution:	Age	36	36–40	41–50	51–60	61
	% of total exams	12%	19%	31%	24%	14%
	% with cancer	1%	3%	25%	36%	35%

Of 5,534 recommendations for biopsy, 3,624 were done and 846 cancer found.

				Negative Axillary Nodes	
	Exams	No. of Ca	Rate/1000	No. of Ca	% of Ca
Initial Exams	70,467	595	8.4	285	48%
Subsequent Exams	92,409	251	2.7	185	74%

On initial exam, the number of prevalent cancers present was high, depending on such factors as self-selection and age of women. Because cancers had been present for varying lengths of time, only half were free of nodal involvement. On subsequent examination the number of incident cancers, which had become detectable since the previous examination was much lower, but the majority had no nodal spread.

found by mammography alone had no nodal involvement, as did 65% of those with cancers found by palpation alone, while 44% of women with cancers found by both methods had negative nodes. The importance of teaching breast self-examination is emphasized by the finding of 9% (or 74) interval cancers with 66% or 49 of them with no nodal involvement.

Breast Cancer Detection Demonstration Projects

With the Guttman Institute as a prototype, 26 other screening projects, involving 28 other centers, have been funded by the National Cancer Institute and the American Cancer Society. About 280,000 women have been involved in this program. The objectives of the program were to demonstrate whether women could be motivated to accept screening and whether substantial numbers of breast cancers could be found in a localized, potentially curable stage. Both objectives have been fulfilled.

The allotted numbers of screenees were rapidly filled in all centers and substantial numbers of early cancers found. Mammography has been found to be particularly effective in detecting early and even minimal cancers. As of early 1977, 2,379 cancers had been found. Of these, 44% were detected on mammography and were not palpable, with 77% having negative nodes. Also, 40% of the cancer were found in women under age 50, and 73% of these women had negative nodes. Women over age 50 and 60% of the cancers, with 79% negative nodes. Comparable figures from the H.I.P. data were 33% of cancers found on x-ray alone, with 79% negative nodes; 23% of

Table II.
Value of the Tandem Technique

The tandem technique, using clinical examination, mammography and thermography gave the highest yield of cancers because some were detectable on only one modality. Those found on one modality only had a higher percentage of negative nodes.

In 972 cancers (excluding 74 "interval" cancers)

Cancers Detected by:	All Cancers		Negative Axillary Nodes	
	No. of Ca	% of Ca	No. of Ca	% of Ca
Mammography only not palpable	155	20%	108	70%
Clinical exam only not on x-ray	170	22%	110	65%
Both felt on palpation and seen on mammogram	447	58%	195	44%

Notes: 1. "Interval" cancers: of the 846 cancers found, 772 were detected on screening modalities and 74 were "interval" cancers found by the women themselves within a year of a negative examination. They were not included in the tally above.

2. Thermography, when abnormal, alerts the physician to the possible presence of cancer in a stage not yet detectable by palpation or mammography and suggests more frequent examinations in order to localize it earlier. Since a positive thermogram alone is never the basis for biopsy, it was also not represented in the data above.

3. Negative nodes were included in the above data only when proven. The surgical procedures in 13% of the cases did not include axillary dissection, so that the true percentage of negative nodes might be higher.

the cancers were in women under age 50 with 68% having negative nodes. Even more important, in the H.I.P. study, 3.5% of the cancers found were under 1 cm in diameter with 58.6% of these found on the x-ray alone.

Apparently, the improved mammographic techniques used in the new studies have resulted in a substantial increase in cancers found on mammography alone, especially in women under age 50 and especially in cancers under 1 cm in size.

Lundgren Swedish Project (Lundgren et al., 1976)

All women aged 40 years and over residing in the county of Gavle (a total of 37,540 women) were invited to a screening program. About 83% responded to the examination, which involved only one oblique projection in mammography. No routine clinical study was made. Those women (366) with positive findings on mammography received palpation. There were five inoperable cancers. Biopsies were done on 207 of the remaining women, in whom 125 carcinomas were found; 22 lesions were considered precancerous and 60 were considered benign. Of the cancer patients 87% had no axillary nodal involvement.

De Waard Holland Project (DeWaard, 1978)

DeWaard and his colleagues surveyed over 14,000 women, aged 50 to 64, with clinical examination and mammography; 253 biopsies were performed and 106 breast cancers found. In the six-month recall group, 15 additional biopsies were performed and four cancers were found. There was no axillary nodal involvement in 66% of the cancers. Only one of the 110 cancers was found on clinical examination alone, while 57% of the cancers were found on mammography alone. Only five "interval" cancers were found.

Apparently the improved techniques available today are resulting in greater mammographic pickup than was noted in the H.I.P. study. New studies are pointing up the increasing value of mammography in screening.

CONCLUSIONS

There is general agreement that the earlier in its cycle a breast cancer is detected and treated, the greater is the likelihood of increased survival and cure. Early detection involves at least three general principles:

1) Since advancing age is the most important risk factor, and since most breast cancer is detectable in women over age 50, and since definite proof in this age group exists that screening for the disease will lower the death rate by at least 40% and that mammography as well as palpation are necessary for such reduction, it is imperative that screening using both modalities become a routine part of the medical examination of all women over age 50 on an annual basis.

2) Since the symptomatic woman with a dominant mass or a persistent pain or nipple discharge may have these symptoms because of an underlying cancer, all such women should have a complete breast examination including mammography or any other diagnostic study as often as is necessary to make sure cancer is or is not present.

3) Mammographic technique used under all circumstances should be the one producing the greatest detail and resolution, with the lowest amount of radiation needed to produce high quality films. The techniques should be subject to change as new knowledge and technology provide improvement in these areas.

Readily available and in use are techniques that deliver doses down to .02 rads to the mid breast. This low dosage can be considered negligible in comparison with the presumed benefit from mammography.

4) All primary care physicians be they gynecologists or generalists must assume the responsibility for screening for breast cancer. They can fulfill that responsibility in three ways:

a) It is the duty of all phsycians to teach breast self-examination (B.S.E.) to every woman, even and especially, those without breast complaints. Of course, physicians must themselves be knowledgeable about the method.

b) It is the duty of all physicians to examine the breasts of his women patients, particularly those over age 30, at the time of any clinical study. Of course, physicians should take the trouble to learn from an expert how to do a good clinical examination.

c) It is the duty of all physicians to encourage all women patients over age 35 to have thorough breast examinations once a year, including, if appropriate, mammography and thermography in addition to the breast clinical examination. Of course, physicians should become aware of the progress that has been made in the detection of early breast cancer using new modalities.

REFERENCES

Bailar, J.C. Mammography - a contrary view. *Ann. Intern. Med.* 84:77, 1976.

Copeland, M.M. The Challenge of Breast Cancer. *Bull. Amer. Coll. Surg.* 63:2, 1978.

Day, E., Venet, L. Periodic cancer detection examinations as a control measure. In Fourth National Cancer Conference Proceedings. Philadelphia, J.B. Lippincott, 1961.

DeWaard, F. Argumenten Voor Bevolksonderzdek or Borstkanker *T. Soc. Geneesk.* 56:9, 1978.

Egan, R.L. Mammography, an aid to diagnosis of breast carcinoma. *J.A.M.A.* 182:938, 1962.

Fink, R., Strax, P., Venet, L. Evaluation of thermography in mass screening for breast cancer. In Proceedings of Third International Symposium of Detection and Prevention of Cancer. Marcel Dekker, New York, 1979.

Friedman, A.K., et al. A cooperative evaluation of mammography in seven teaching hospitals. *Radiology* 86:886, 1966.

Gershon-Cohen, J., Hermel, M.B., Berger, S.M. Detection of breast cancer by periodiic x-ray examination. *J.A.M.A.* 176:1114, 1961.

Gilbertsen, W.A., Kfelsberg, I.M. Detection of breast cancer by periodic utilization of methods of physical diagnosis. *Cancer* 28:1552, 1971.

Holleb, A.I., Venet, L., Day, E., Hoyt, S. Breast cancer detected by routine physical examinations. *N.Y. State J. Med.* 60:823, 1960.

Isard, H.J., Ostrum, B.J. Breast thermography — the mammatherm. *Radiol. Clin. North. Am.* 12:167, 1974.

Lawson, R.N. Implications of the surface temperatures in the diagnosis of breast cancer. *Can. Med. Assoc. J.* 75:309, 1956.

Lundgren, B., Jakobssen, S. Single view mammography in breast cancer screening *Cancer* 38:1124, 1976.

Miller, D.W., Hammerstein, G.R., White, Dr., et al. Radiation absorbed dose in mammography. Presented at annual meeting of Amer. Assoc. of Physicists in Medicine, Cincinnati, 1977.

Moskowitz, M. et al. Lack of efficacy of thermography as a screening tool for minimal and stage 1 breast cancer *New Eng. J. Med.* 295:249, 1976.

Ostrum, B.J., Becker, W., Isard, H.J. Low dose mammography. *Radiology* 190:323, 1973.

Price, J.L., Nathan, B.L. Radiological aspects of the West London screening program for breast neoplasms. *Proc R. Soc. Med.* 68:438, 1975.

Shapiro, S., Strax, P., Venet, L., Venet, W. Changes in 5 year breast cancer screening program. In Proceedings of Seventh National Cancer Conference. Philadelphia: J. B. Lippincott, 1973.

Stevens, G.M., Weigen, J.F. Mammography screening for breast cancer detection. *Cancer* 19:51, 1966.

Strax, P. Breast cancer diagnosis: Mammography, thermography and xerography: A commentary. *J. Reprod. Med.* 4:265, 1975.

Strax, P. Benefit of breast cancer screening on morbidity and mortality. In Skandia International Sumposia, Health Control in Detection of Cancer. Stockholm: Almqvist and Almqvist Wiksell Internat., 1976.

Strax, P. Control of breast cancer through mass screening in breast cancer. New York: Alan R. Liss, 1977.

Venet, L., Strax, P., Venet, W., Shapiro, S. Adequacies and inadequacies of breast examinations by physicians in mass screening. *Cancer* 28:1546, 1971.

Wilkinson, E., Jacobson, G., Montz, E.P. Preliminary clinical mammography study using electron radiography. In Proceedings of Third International Symposium of Detection and Prevention of Cancer. New York: Marcel Dekker.   1979.

Wolfe, J.N. Xeroradiography of the breast. Springfield, Ill.: Charles C Thomas, 1972.

CHAPTER 4

Gynecological Management in Breast Malignancy

ROBERT C. WALLACH

Although the direct surgical involvement of obstetrician-gynecologists in the management of breast disease has long ago been handed over to the surgeons who specialize in this area, the involvement of the obstetrician-gynecologist in the total management of breast disease continues to be most important. The gynecologist has increasingly assumed the role of the primary physician to women in addition to providing specialized surgical skills for the problems of the female reproductive system. The primary care role of the gynecologist gives him or her access to female patients at all stages in their reproductive spans and at all ages in their lives. For many women, the gynecologist is the central focus of medical care and the routine gynecologic examination is the only dependable, repetitive contact with organized health care. This dependence on the gynecologist places a burden on him or her to provide screening and referral services for *all* types of medical problems but, especially for the related areas of breast and endocrine problems, the patient will expect the gynecologist to maintain a level of expertise and provide access to appropriate care when indicated.

HISTORY

History-taking for the gynecologist requires attention to those factors in both the personal and family background that may delineate the patient at increased risk for breast cancer. Inquiry into the incidence of breast cancer in the family is crucial, since this disease is frequently seen in multiple members of the family unit. With decreasing size of individual family units, the availability of this type of information will probably diminish over the years, but it is always worthwhile to review the experience of the patient's mother, aunts, sisters, and other bloodline relatives.

In addition, the history of other malignancies in the family may bear on the future prospects of the individual patient. Associations have been noted between breast cancer and genital tract malignancy, although the relatively high frequency of these diseases in our society clouds the issue of common cause and exposure. Benign disease of the breast in the patient or in the family is worthy of note, although the relation to the subsequent onset of malignant disease has not been established. A history of cystic mastitis, or fibrocystic disease (or similar descriptions for this entity), will attract attention to the patient's physical examination although here too, a predisposition to malignancy has not been established. A major problem exists in the difficulty of physical examination when cystic mastitis is present, as the small malignant neoplasm may be obscured by the thickened cords of breast tissue.

Other items of personal history that may prove relevant in years to come are exposure to diagnostic or therapeutic x-ray, chemical carcinogen exposure, hormonal treatment, or long-term treatment with medication which might alter the susceptibility to breast malignancy.

An apparent increasing frequency in cosmetic breast surgery will also attract attention to those patients who have had either reductive or augmentative mammoplasty, since in these patients the physical examination will be difficult. It is unlikely that surgical scars will predispose these patients to the induction of mammary cancer, but they will undoubtedly provide difficulty in interpretation of physical findings. Currently, the prostheses used for augmentation mammoplasty are made of inert substances that generally do not have direct access to cell physiology and therefore would not be anticipated to provide carcinogenic stimulus. But the long-term application of a foreign body, however bland, may be synergistic with other influences in the induction of breast cancer, although this has never been found in clinical experience. The diffuse injection of substances such as silicone for breast augmentation has passed out of popularity, although many women who have had these procedures will be available for examination and should be the subject of the closest scrutiny.

Requests for advice about availabilties, and indications for mammoplasty, reduction or augmentations, are common. Sometimes, the obstetrician-gynecologist will have an insight into the patient's emotional make-up that will help in guiding her decision. Many patients will first voice concerns about breast size to the gynecologist who must evaluate the need and make available competent plastic surgery consultation. Pregnancy after cosmetic breast surgery is generally not a problem, although mammoplasty frequently obviates the possibility of breast-feeding.

ORAL CONTRACEPTIVES

A major subject of concern for the gynecologist is the administration of oral contraceptives. In a relatively short period of time, the introduction of oral contraceptives has made a major impact in most industrial societies. Within the last 20 years the availability of effective oral contraception has led to its acceptance and widespread use, and only in recent years have serious questions been raised concerning the safety of these potent agents. Perhaps never before have so many human beings been treated with such effective systemic medication in the absence of the formal elements of disease as evidenced by local pathology. The increasing fertility rate as a reflection of control of various disease factors, changes in population related to the reduction of childhood disease, and improved sanitation measures have made the oral contraceptive a major factor in both individual lives and in the population control plans of nations.

In a relatively short period of time, also, the contraceptive drugs and the dosages of these drugs have undergone modifications and there has been a disturbing lack of prospective and retrospective studies on the potential for problems of these oral contraceptives. In just a few years the dosage of oral contraceptives has changed from that of the initial pills, which was in the range of 10 mg of a potent synthetic progestagen (19 nor-steriods) with a concomitant synthetic estrogen, to the current pills which frequently have 1 mg or 0.5 mg of a progestagen and occasionally a higher dose of the synthetic estrogen.

Comparisons of the pharmacologic activity of the various preparations have usually relied heavily on selected animal studies, which lend themselves to quantification. In the human subject, however, the anticipated variety of response makes such comparison in inbred animal colonies of limited value. The primary effects of oral contraceptives are on the pituitary, which is suppressed, the endometrium, whose growth pattern is altered, and the cervix, whose mucus is modified. These effects lead to anovulation and the inability of the uterus to promote and accept conception.

Clinical effects of contraceptive drugs on the breasts have been frequently noted, although dependable data are lacking. It is, for instance, unknown at this time what the effects of the various estrogen compounds available are on breast tissue, and it is also unknown whether these effects are controlled or altered by the synthetic progestagens given in association. Patients will frequently report a difference in breast size, shape, and sensitivity while using oral contraceptives, and these changes will frequently mimic pregnancy effects. Water retention in breast tissue is thought to be a major factor in these changes, although little information is available concerning the changes in the stroma of these organs.

Important questions are raised with the use of oral contraceptives. Does the long-term use of estrogen in cyclic fashion lead to the induction of breast carcinoma? If the long-term use of estrogen does not itself induce breast carcinoma, what is its effect on the woman who is predisposed to breast carcinoma for other reasons? Will she have her disease earlier, with more aggressive malignancy, or other altered biology? Does the progestagen that may confer effects related to those of pregnancy provide any measure of protection for either the patient at high risk or for the average woman? What is the significance of the varying combinations of drugs available, whether these be standard dose, low dose, microdose, or progestagen-only compounds? Is there an ideal dose combination to minimize the carcinogenic stimulus to the breast? The answers to *none* of these questions are available at this time. Prospective studies are desirable, but the author is unaware of any along these lines.

Because of the relatively short exposure of the population to these drugs, any effect which might be exerted has not yet had an opportunity to be expressed. On the other hand, increasing reports of varying validity concerning other hazards of oral contraceptives continue to fill both the scientific journals and the lay press. The hazards of thrombophlebitis, pulmonary embolism, hypertension, cerebrovascular accidents, early coronary disease, liver tumors, etc. provide scare-reading in magazines directed at women and in otherwise dry issues of the daily newspapaers.

The relation of oral contraceptives to the breast has not attracted enough medical attention, although the breast is responsive to these hormones. It is also unclear whether women with a family history of breast malignancy should be considered candidates for oral contraceptives or whether they should be advised against their use. The general conservative attitude of physicians would probably advise against the use of oral contraceptives or any hormones in the woman whose family history suggests hormone-sensitive tumors.

ESTROGEN REPLACEMENT

Within the last few years enormous attention has been directed toward the use of estrogen replacement, which has been practical and popular in the U.S. since just before the start of the Second World War. Although one well-known preparation of conjugated estrogens has dominated the market, there is available a host of preparations of purely estrogenic substances generally given to menopausal women who complain of the symptoms related to estrogen withdrawal—vasomotor instability (hot flushes), vaginal dryness, irritability, depression, etc.

The use of estrogen replacement for its possible help in the control of coronary disease has attracted much speculation but here, too, dependable studies are lacking. Aggravation of coronary disease in men treated with estrogens for prostatic carcinoma has been reported, but it is unclear whether there is an analogy from this for women patients.

The use of estrogens for the prevention of osteoporosis or its subsequent control has also led to confusing statements and treatment plans offered to women patients. Recent highly publicized studies concerning the relation of estrogen replacement and the induction of endometrial carcinoma have tended to substantiate the known relation between unopposed estrogen, endometrial hyperplasia, and carcinoma, which was reported many years ago in women. Analogous studies in animals are not very useful because of species differences and end organ differences.

Although not universally applicable, sampling techniques for endometrium, when feasible, have provided a measure of security regarding the use of estrogen in menopausal women. Unfortunately, no such technique is available for evaluation of the effect on the breast, if there is, indeed, a relationship. Various treatment plans for menopausal symptoms have been advocated, and generally these are a reflection of the concern for the effect on the endometrium. In the past, estrogen medication was given on a daily basis at a predetermined dose. This dose would be established by arbitrarily selecting and maintaining one, beginning with a low dose and raising it until symptoms were controlled, or by beginning with a high dose and reducing it until symptoms reappeared. In order to avoid the effects of unopposed estrogen and the possible induction of endometrial hyperplasia, estrogens have been given in a cycle with five or seven days in each calendar month reserved for no medication. More recently the addition of a potent oral progestagen to either cyclic or continuous estrogen administration has received wide popularity and increasing acceptance.

Although the primary concern in the administration of these drugs has been focused on the endometrium, the potential for an effect on the breast remains to be seen. In the case of patients with established breast malignancy, whether controlled or uncontrolled, the use of hormones should be predicated on the treatment plan for the breast cancer rather than for the amelioration of menopausal symptoms. Drugs aimed at the control of autonomic nervous system instability, generally belladonna alkaloids and others, may frequently be used with either potential or established breast malignancy without invoking the known or suspected problem of the hormones.

EPIDEMIOLOGICAL FACTORS

In the role of obstetrician, many physicians will be questioned concerning the known epidemiologic relation between childbirth and breast-feeding and breast cancer. It is apparent that in large groups of women whose initial childbearing occurs at relatively young ages and for whom larger families are the rule, breast cancer is less common than for those women whose childbearing is less frequent and starts later. The associated socioeconomic factors are difficult to dissociate but the relation seems well established. There are very few women whose plans for childbearing will be predicated on the prophylaxis of breast carcinoma, but this information should be disseminated as part of the educational responsibility of the obstetrician-gynecologist.

Breast-feeding, likewise, has an apparently protective effect against the subsequent origin of breast cancer. Whether this effect is from the breast feeding process itself or from the reflex change in the hormonal pattern of the woman with sustained low estrogen effects and progestagen dominance is unclear. The recent trend toward the popularity of breast feeding is a complex sociologic phenomenon but may exert some salutary effect on the subsequent incidence of breast cancer. This must, however, be balanced against a lowered birthrate and a tendency to later onset of childbearing in many families, especially in the urban environment.

BREAST EXAMINATIONS

The obstetrician-gynecologist will frequently bear the responsibility for being the sole physician available for breast examination. The usual timing of such an examination is determined by the preference and training of the physician. Frequently the scheduling of the "annual" check-up and Pap smear have determined the frequency of breast examination. For those patients with particular gynecological problems or pregnancy, more frequent examination for those reasons may provide greater access to breast examination.

It goes without saying that each gynecologic examination must include the competent examination of the breasts. Some obstetrician-gynecologists increase the frequency of examinations of women in the perimenopausal years because of the increased likelihood of gynecologic problems at that time. Frequent examinations of women in the age range with a greater incidence of breast carcinoma will provide a greater access to physical diagnosis at an early stage. The breast exam should never be left out regardless of the frequency or repetitive nature of examinations by the gynecologist.

For example, occasional patients will be seen who call attention to some particular part of their examination and the complete examination is not done for months or years. Although the pregnant patient is generally in an age range carrying less than maximal risk for breast carcinoma, the breast examination must be included. It is unfortunate that following the initial obstetric examination the breast examination is frequently overlooked until the patient's postpartum visit. Dr. Louis Hellman, Once commenting on the case of a breast carcinoma that arose during pregnancy after a negative initial exam by a competent examiner, suggested that the breast exam be repeated as a standard procedure in the month prior to delivery. Clearly, the engorgement and hormonal effects of the breasts in pregnancy make the examination more difficult.

An issue that has attracted wide publicity and is currently unresolved is the appropriate time for the initial referral and subsequent referrals for screening mammography. The risk of x-ray-induced carcinoma of the breast has been widely publicized on the basis of both the theoretical hazard and the known incidence of malignancy in survivors of the Hiroshima and Nagasaki bombing. Questionable results of studies of those patients exposed to diganostic mammography in previous years have also been widely discussed. Without resolution many factors must be considered in the individual decision for screening mammography. Whether the patient is in a high-risk category should be determined and, if so, the theoretical risks are probably less important than the practical advantage of dependable screening.

The appropriate age for the initial mammography is in itself a very complex issue. In young women during the reproductive years the physiologic activity of the breast makes for a more difficult physical examination as well as mammographic examination; there is the technical difficulty of interpreting the results. This has been used as an argument to defer mammography until the perimenopausal years, when the ease of pick-up of small lesions is greater. The philosophical arguments about where weight should be given in this discussion are beyond the scope of this presentation. It should, however, be stressed that in families in which breast carcinoma has arisen early in the family history, individual patients will probably do well to have mammography performed at appropriate ages.

Appropriate intervals for repeat mammography have not been established. The highest frequency of referral for screening mammography will probably be at a yearly interval although alternate yearly intervals have achieved some popularity. Whether the total dose is a factor in the subsequent induction of malignancy has yet to be established although this is felt to be a theoretical possibility. It has not been determined whether there is a minimal threshold dose below which no malignancy can be induced and up to which mammography could be used safely. This awaits unstarted studies in the radiobiology of this situation. If there is a carcinogenic influence of mammography, and if the generally accepted two-decade latent period for the induction of human malignancy applies, it may be that there is a trade-off for the perimenopausal woman between the early detection of breast carcinoma in those years and the subsequent development of this same malignancy in later years. Comparison of the malignancy and outcome for radiation-induced breast malignancy and other malignancies of the breast is unavailable.

Very frequently abnormalities in the breast tissue will be discovered by the patient herself. On the other hand, it is only in recent years that breast self-examination has achieved any wide popularity. Instruction in breast self-examination can easily be given in a short period of time in a doctor's office; educational material is available for patient and physician. In the usual course of events of harried and hectic and over-booked private practice and clinic situations, however, individual patient education by physicians frequently suffers. An alternative to this is to have a physician's assistant, nurse, or nurse's aide adequately instructed in the techniques of breast self-examination so that she may help the physician by providing instruction for the patient. The reaction of many patients to breast self-examination is a positive interest in their own welfare but some women become anxious about this instruction and shy away from it.

SURGERY

Even though the obstetrician-gynecologist has long ago abandoned his role in the primary surgical management of breast disease, there are occasionally places where he may be of service. The role of the obstetrician-gynecologist in the aspiration of cystic masses of the breast depends on local conduct of this situation, and the standard of practice in the community will determine whether the obstetrician-gynecologist should do this procedure.

One of the major functions of the gynecologist in the management of breast malignancy is in his contribution to ablative surgery for established or disseminated breast carcinoma. For those breast malignancies known or suspected to be estrogen-sensitive, the removal of functioning ovaries may frequently provide a measure of relief and form a major part of the therapeutic plan. In addition, the ovary is very frequently the site of metastasis of breast carcinoma, even in the absence of established metastases elsewhere. In these cases, the gynecologist will frequently be called upon to do a bilateral oophorectomy. The procedure of choice will frequently be a total abdominal hysterectomy and bilateral salpingo-oophorectomy.

In patients at low risk for cervical carcinoma and for whom the life expectancy from their disseminated breast malignancy is small, even the few minutes necessary for removal of the cervix at the time of ablative surgery may not be justified and a supracervical hysterectomy may be combined with bilateral salpingo-oophorectomy in these patients. Occasionally, for technical reasons, the procedure of choice may be bilateral salpingo-oophorectomy alone with conservation of the uterus. This would be the case most commonly in the occasional patient who is a poor medical risk and for whom there is great mobility of the ovaries because of a long utero-ovarian ligament, which provides easy access to the ovaries without interference or manipulation of the uterus.

These decisions will be made at the time of surgery, but if the uterus is to be left behind an endometrial sample must be obtained, preferably in advance, as this is occasionally the site for metastasis of breast carcinoma or of a separate malignancy. Any patient under observation for breast malignancy, whether controlled or disseminated, should have frequent and regular pelvic examinations for detection of ovarian enlargement, both on the basis of possible metastasis or of a separate primary carcinoma. The relation of breast and ovarian carcinoma has been established and should not be overlooked.

Prophylactic oophorectomy has largely been superseded in the management of breast carcinoma by the cautious advocacy of therapeutic removal of the ovaries only in an established estrogen-dependent breast carcinoma with signs of dissemination. Occasionally with determination of estrogen receptors in a young patient at high risk for dissemination, early or prophylactic removal of the ovaries may be warranted. Clearly, in this situation estrogen replacement for menopausal symptoms induced by ovarian removal cannot be used, and control of autonomic nervous system symptoms will be a goal of treatment.

A major responsibility of the gynecologist is to establish referral patterns for consultation on abnormal findings in breast disease, for evaluation of mammography, and for hospitalization and treatment of patients with disseminated breast malignancy. It is the responsibility of the obstetrician-gynecologist to be aware of the physicians in his community who have special expertise in breast cancer and who can provide the best care for referred patients. The obstetrician-gynecologist must also stay conversant with major trends in treatment in order to provide useful counselling to these patients, who will frequently return for professional support during the stressful times related to their breast cancer.

CHAPTER 5

Some Psychiatric Aspects Of Mastectomy

MAX NEEDLEMAN

It is my purpose, in this chapter, to discuss some psychiatric factors sur-rounding the procedure of mastectomy for cancer of the breast, which have not been given sufficient attention in the past. It is suggested that further in-vestigation and study of such areas could be useful in furthering the reduc-tion of the emotional and mental disturbances that can and do result from such surgery and in limiting its traumatic consequences.

One must keep in mind that in order to fully understand the reactions, the needs, fears, and wishes of our patient, both conscious and unconscious fields of influence should be examined, if possible. Clinical experience teaches us that depressed feelings and attitudes may be responsible for emotional sequelae, prolonged reactions, and disturbed behavior. Too often, neglect of this information can have unfortunate and lifelong results (Harrell, 1972). Making such information available to those who are in-volved in the treatment of the patient, or to the family, and to the patient herself, makes more possible a more complete rehabilitation—both surgical and emotional—which is so important to the enhancement of the quality of life (Markel, 1971).

The emotional reactions, sequelae, and complications of women exposed to this traumatic surgery must not be underestimated or minimized. Life it-self, even when not curtailed, may be seriously impaired by the possible loss of desire for participation, the development of a dependency on drugs and alcohol, and finally, by impulses for suicide, when psychological factors are unrecognized or ignored (Ervin, 1973).

Fortunately, however, there has been a gratifying growing awareness of the fact that women who have mastectomies may be traumatized emotion-ally or mentally. It is recognized that these women must deal with many psychological problems, in one way or another, both preoperatively and postoperatively.

The reaction to this tragic development in a woman's life is inevitably highly individualized. The reaction may be mild or severe; it can be brief or permanent. Much depends on individual character or personality structure. The response is related to the intensity of the woman's fears of loss of sexual attractiveness and of fears of rejection. Her reaction will depend on whether she feels irreversibly mutilated, crippled, and repulsive. Much of it will depend on her previous history and style of life, on her ability to cope with acute loss and deprivation, and on other psychic traumata in her earlier life.

PREPARATION FOR MASTECTOMY

There is general acceptance of the idea that adequate preoperative preparation, both medical and psychological, is useful in reducing the trauma of surgery and its postoperative sequelae. Preoperative discussions and communication with the patient for the purposes of verbalizing and exposing her fears, anxieties, and fantasies in anticipating surgery has been found to be psychologically beneficial in modifying attitudes and subsequently in reducing postoperative psychiatric difficulties.

This procedure has been effective in preparing children for major or minor surgery (including tonsillectomy), when we can expect significant psychological reactions. Such preparation has been used, with benefit, prior to hysterectomy, amputation, and other major procedures. It is well-known that the incidence of postoperative psychiatric sequelae in emergency surgery which allows no time for the opportunity for preparation and discussion, is much higher than that of elective surgery which does allow time and opportunity for such preparation. Literature documents the fact that psychiatric preparation and counselling prior to cardiac surgery has reduced the incidence of postoperative psychiatric complications signficantly. One may compare this procedure to the similar, accepted medical principle of permitting the development of adequate immunologic defenses before exposure to infection or antigen.

It is the experience of many psychiatrists who are asked to see women preoperatively, i.e., prior to biopsy, for the prupose of preparing such patients for mastectomy, that the effort was generally ineffective. Since there was no definite proof of malignancy, at that point, but only a possibility or probability (as is always true before biopsy) the patient could not permit herself to focus on the possible malignancy and mastectomy, but found herself concentrating obsessively on the persistent and natural wishes that the tumor would turn out to be benign and that there would be no loss of a breast—all of this in spite of frightening thoughts and fantasies.

It is because of these experiences, and because of the experiences in other surgical situations mentioned above, that the routine surgical consent requirement, which asks that women sign permission forms for biopsy and at the same time for mastectomy, is being seriously questioned. This routine requirement is considered to be psychologically unsound and not in the best interests of good patient care.

It is my belief that, with this routine procedure, the patient cannot be expected to prepare herself adequately, with suitable defenses, for the loss of a breast. With such a routine procedure, the patient enters the operating room and is put under anesthesia, never knowing definitely, despite repeated warnings, whether she has cancer and whether her breast will be removed. As long as there is no definite proof of cancer (and there rarely is prior to biopsy), that patient will concentrate on the natural wish that the tumor will turn out to be benign and that there will be no loss of the breast.

The patient cannot be expected to deal with a possibility or probability; she has a much better chance to cope with, and to make her adjustment to, a *reality*. But with the above routine method, the existence of cancer and the loss of a breast becomes a reality to her only when she awakens in the recovery room minus the breast, before she has been able to psychologically prepare herself for this horrendous loss. And it is because of this unpreparedness that the woman frequently is left with doubt as to whether the mastectomy was really necessary, and with feelings of anger and resentment.

There is, no doubt, reasonable surgical justification for the procedure that has been followed for many years, including the avoidance of giving anesthesia twice. It is also quite understandable that the patient herself would generally go along with this routine procedure, and even prefer to avoid making two decisions requiring two signatures. And certainly the patient generally would prefer to avoid that period of waiting and of worry, which would be inevitable if she had to sign for mastectomy after biopsy—i.e., after the diagnosis had been made.

But, from the psychological point of view, it is a mistake to encourage or, in fact, to permit the patient to avoid this second period of worry or preparation. This is the period when the patient would face the actual fact of the diagnosis of cancer, which would then make it more possible for her to mobilize her defenses and to become psychologically prepared for this most difficult event.

It is for these reasons that the recommendation is made that, in most instances, patients should be asked to sign for mastectomy only after the pathological diagnosis has been established by biopsy, and that patients should be encouraged to endure a short interval between operations because it is psychologically advisable and in their long-range interests. Many postoperative emotional reactions including anger, rage, depression, suspicion, and bitterness, the incidence of which is greater than we realize, could frequently be avoided. This interval between operations could be used with benefit for support and counselling by family, surgeon, social worker, and by psychiatrist.

SURGICAL AND PSYCHOLOGICAL REHABILITATION

There is a continuing interest in the rehabilitation of the woman who has lost a breast, not only from the surgical but also from the psychological point of view. There is a derservedly and understandably persistent effort to improve the quality of these women's lives. To further these objectives, reconstruction and replacement of the breast are the subjects of much study and have been receiving increasing attention both in the professional literature and in the media. It seems, however, that much of the impetus for the development of this type of rehabilitation and the push for its acceptance as a useful and necessary follow-up procedure of mastectomy have come more from efforts of women who have either benefited from, or have been deprived of, this plastic repair than from the medical professionals. More interest in and committment to this rehabilitative effort might develop among physicians and surgeons if they realized that the psychological benefits derived from reconstruction, in addition to the improved cosmetic appearance it creates, are very significant and that such procedures whenever possible, would be important in more ways than meet the eye.

The impetus for reconstruction of the breast that surgeons have emphasized has been derived from their wish to restore the body image usually for young women who are considered to be interested in clothes, bathing suits, and for women who continue to have an interest in an active sex life. Surgeons have considered and recommended this repair for women who have been especially concerned with appearance or for those who may have felt particularly mutilated or repulsive by the loss of the breast. This approach tended to limit this procedure to only a certain group of women, a narrow segment of those who have lost breasts.

There should be increasing recognition of the fact that so-called older women continue to have an interest in an active sex life and the need to feel complete and attractive. Older women may have these continuing needs and wishes but might be reluctant to admit to such "unimportant" or "frivolous" interests. Clinical experience suggests that some older women resign themselves to the deprivation and to the mutilation because of feelings of guilt and because they consider it "inappropriate" to admit to the continuing need for such gratifications. This becomes a resignation or settling procedure which leads to an impaired and deprived existence, which should be neither necessary nor encouraged.

Perhaps such attitudes on the part of some older patients are compounded and solidified by the attitudes of some physicians and surgeons. Thus, physicians may believe that older people have given up sex and no longer require sexual gratification. In fact, such physicians may feel that older people should no longer be interested in sex and attractiveness.

The comment of the surgeon to the woman past age fifty who has had a mastectomy—"You're lucky because you don't have to worry about that anymore"—is reported from time to time. But, there is clinical evidence and psychological proof to suggest that sexual needs continue for most people in older life, and that therefore the quality of life for older women who have had mastectomies would be importantly enhanced by reconstruction and replacement of the breast, if possible. Jean Zalon (Zalon, 1978), in a recently published book, makes the statement, "What good does it do to save a woman's life and then condemn her to a life she hardly finds worth living?"

The following are accounts of the experiences of three women who had reconstructive surgery, with replacement of the breast. The first is a 57-year-old woman who was not aware of the possibility of replacement prior to mastectomy; the second is a 33-year-old woman with whom replacement of the breast was discussed and arranged for prior to mastectomy. The third interview was held with a young woman of 33 who had demanded an interval between the biopsy and mastectomy, and who was fully aware of the breast replacement procedure.

Patient A:

Dr.: We are interested in understanding your thoughts and feelings with respect to the replacement of your breast by reconstructive surgery; we are interested in your opinion as to its cosmetic advantages, but also how you view its psychological usefulness or necessity.

Pt.: For me, the results of replacement of the breast was quite miraculous. When I first asked for it, everyone thought I was on a vanity trip, a request which was not becoming to a woman of my age.

Dr.: When did you have this reconstruction?

Pt.: Three and a half years after the mastectomy.

Dr.: In your opinion, would it have been useful to know about reconstruction before mastectomy?

Pt.: Tremendously. Following mastectomy, there was a feeling of being less feminine; my body was very unattractive to me; I felt that every man would think of me as repulsive. The reconstruction made me feel whole again. But to answer your question, if I had known about replacement before mastectomy, I would have gone into the original surgery with much less sadness and with more hope. In fact, the loss of the breast seemed to me to be the immediate response; the fear of cancer and death was, at the beginning, secondary. Every time I looked at that area and that scar, I had a constant reminder of cancer. The replacement of the breast began to make me feel, gradually, only remotely related to cancer. This was in addition to the fact that it contributed to an ease of living, with less concern about clothes, bathing suits, etc.

Dr.: Has reconstruction helped you in your sexual activities and in the general relationship with men?

Pt.: Yes. I am more fond of my body. I don't feel that I will repel anybody. I am more free. Before reconstruction, I was reluctant to show my body, and literally always tried to cover that area; I wouldn't allow anyone to see it. I am at ease now in revealing my body.

Dr.: Would you consider yourself to be a woman who is particularly concerned about body and appearance, and about feeling complete?

Pt.: Not at all. I don't believe I am particularly vain. I believe that this is how all women would feel, with the sense of being whole.

Dr.: How did you learn about reconstruction?

Pt.: A young woman dermatologist asked me, "Why are you walking around like this—it's ridiculous."

Dr.: When did you learn about having cancer?

Pt.: It was six years ago—and I reacted with disbelief and with feelings of anger and fury with my family, my doctor, and with the world. If I had been told then that I could live a normal life and could participate in all activities, I would have been more hopeful, less angry, and more accepting of the original surgery.

Dr.: Having had reconstructive surgery, how would you evaluate and summarize the results?

Pt.: It has helped me to avoid an enormous amount of suffering and anguish. And now I can go about my business and live my life—and not be uncomfortable or concerned. It makes the difference between a partial, unhappy life and a full and happy one.

Patient B:

Dr.: Did you know about the possibility of reconstruction before your mastectomy?

Pt.: No, I first learned about it when the surgeon, who recommended mastectomy, told me immediately that this was a possibility—that I could choose.

Dr.: Did you find it to be a helpful recommendation?

Pt.: It was very helpful. I found it reassuring to talk to the plastic surgeon before mastectomy. It made me feel optimistic, and I felt that there was a promise of a future for me.

Dr.: When you had the mastectomy, what were you concerned about most?

Pt.: My immediate and most intense concern was about mutilation. The fear of cancer and the possible interruption of my life was secondary. Actually, I was really never sure how replacement would work and whether it would be successful, but I felt that the mutilation and the scar would be disgusting and intolerable to me, and so the promise of replacement made me feel more hopeful. I was fearful of the asymmetry which would result from the mastectomy, but even more afraid of the scar.

Dr.: Did you have any preoccupation with fears of loss of femininity?

Pt.: Yes, but with the promise of reconstruction I rapidly developed a hope that I, and other people, could again look at my body without disgust. But I would hardly believe that I could look attractive and sexy again.

Dr.: Suppose reconstruction would not have been possible—what then?

Pt.: I suppose I would have survived. Actually, the scar and mutilation was not as horrible as I expected, but perhaps I was able to accept the scar and mutilation more easily since I knew it was only going to be temporary. This made it more tolerable.

Dr.: Was reconstruction of the breast helpful in adjusting to cancer?

Pt.: Absolutely. Before reconstruction, I was constantly reminded, visually, about it. Once the reconstruction began, I began to forget about cancer and about ever having had it .... I have to tell you that since replacement of the breast, I had an opportunity to go "skinny-dipping" which I had enjoyed many times before this whole business started .... I found myself crying because I was so grateful, and it seemed so incredible to me that I could do it again .... I sometimes have to remind myself that "I was a cancer victim." It doesn't seem to apply to me anymore .... I never worry about getting dressed anymore. I can do it without thinking about it .... I can go braless again just as I had done prior to mastectomy .... After my mastectomy I started to sleep in a nightgown or bathrobe, which was unusual for me. I did this even when I was alone and for some reason or another, I still do it occasionally .... but I feel my body is back together again. It feels natural and normal, which is a feeling that I thought I would never again experience. I feel almost as good as new .... the breast has always been an erogenous zone for me, but having been small-breasted, I was never very eager to be looked at. But now, for some reason, I don't feel that way. I am less sensitive about being looked at and certainly my breast is more sensitive than I expected it to be .... This is a peculiar thing to say, but it seems to me that the worst thing that has ever happened to me (the mastectomy) was associated with the best thing that ever happened to me—the fact that I was able to have the reconstruction surgery. Since I had to have that awful thing happen to me, it was a blessing to have reconstruction . . . . I really feel that it was very helpful that I was told early about reconstruction, that I saw the plastic surgeon before mastectomy. It seems as if it was my lifeline to the future. I really don't understand why doctors hesitate to recommend this to all women . . . . I feel extremely lucky, considering how it all turned out. It seems I was lucky to get the right surgeon, and going to the plastic surgeon was a lifesaver to me . . . . Before reconstruction, I had begun to wonder and to have doubts as to whether I really had to lose my breast, whether I could have had some other form of treatment which some surgeons recommend, and I was beginning to feel somewhat resentful and angry about the loss. But since reconstruction, I have never again had that feeling. I feel so strongly and positive about that experience and I am grateful that my doctor, that is, my surgeon, made it easy and possible for me.

Patient C:

Patient is divorced with two young daughters, ages four and seven.

The patient had known about the possibility of replacement of the breast much before her surgery. She learned about the procedure from her reading.

When told about the possibility that her "lump" was malignant, she was most preoccupied with and most shocked by the idea of her mutilation and loss of femininity. The idea of cancer or death was clearly a secondary consideration and worry. She quickly asked to see a plastic surgeon in order to talk about reconstruction as soon as she learned that she would require mastectomy; she wanted to see illustrations of her finished, replaced breast.

In fact, she was one of those few women who independently requested two operations—one for biopsy, and one for mastectomy, with an interval between the two operations so that she could then arrange for reconstruction. She felt that she wanted time to think about mastectomy after she was sure that her lesion was malignant. She was, from the beginning, sure that she did not want to come out of anesthesia, after surgery, not knowing whether her breast was still there or had been removed. She instinctively knew that she needed time to prepare for the actual decision about mastectomy. She compared it to her divorce. She was unable to prepare for this trauma until she was convinced that it was actually going to take place. She refused, at first, to accept it as a possibility—but once she realized that it was inevitable, she took realistic steps to prepare herself and to cope with it.

The existence of the scars still makes it difficult for her to adjust to the idea of cancer, but she is sure that the absence of the breast would have made it more difficult. She can look at that area now with pleasure and permit her young children to see her undressed, and she feels sure that sexual activity with a man will not be difficult. She is happy that she feels complete and is able to dress comfortably and easily in evening gowns and bathing suits.

There is another important psychological argument for reconstruction of the breast after mastectomy in as many women as possible. This argument, with its psychological justification, would apply to all women, young and old, and even in fact to those women who have no special preoccupation with body image or appearance.

Adequate rehabilitation requires women to make reasonable adjustments to the loss of the breast and to the existence of cancer. These women must become more comfortable with the idea of having cancer and eventually should begin to think in terms of "having had," cancer. If these women are to become less obsessively preoccupied with the cancer in their body, less anxious about recurrences and death, they must begin the process of "forgetting," which can be accomplished gradually by using denial of the idea of illness and cancer, and by suppressing and repressing anxious preoccupations and fantasies. If they are successful with this process, it becomes possible to focus attention on activities and problems separate from illness and permits a more active participation in life.

Unfortunately, however, the visible evidence of the absence of the breast, the visible disfigurement, serves as a repetitive and constant reminder of illness and cancer. Such reminders interfere very seriously with the attempted use of denial and repression, making it either very difficult or, in fact, impossible to give up the preoccupation with its accompanying morbid thoughts. Too often this constant thinking about cancer, generated by daily visual stimulation, encourages avoidance of and withdrawal from relationships; necessitates, at times, the use of tranquilizers and alcohol to mitigate the anguish. All of this inevitably leads to limited living.

Replacement of the breast, therefore, with removal of the visual reminder of illness, permits the effective use of these normal and necessary defenses; it permits these women to "forget" and to eventually adjust to the loss of the breast.

Therefore, it is strongly recommended that reconstructive surgery should be made available to as many women as possible, young and old, in order to make their lives more comfortable, more gratifying, and improved in quality. It is further suggested that women who are facing, or who have had, mastectomies should be informed of reconstruction early and should be encouraged to proceed with this surgery as soon as it is feasible.

PSYCHOSOMATIC CONSIDERATIONS

There has been increasing interest and concern about the existence of both emotional and organic illnesses in the same individual at the same time. The possibility that such concurrent illnesses will inter-react and will destructively influence each other through psychosomatic mechanisms is being taken more seriously by both research and clinical professionals.

We have generally recognized that the emotionally or mentally ill woman who develops a malignancy of the breast and requires mastectomy is faced with the possibility that there will be aggravation or exacerbation of that pre-existing emotional or mental disturbance. Women who are in remission from mental illness can suffer recurrence and rekindling of acute episodes as the result of the stress and anxiety related to the new organic illness requiring surgery. Recurrences of depressions and phobias, which have been clinically observed repeatedly, result in severe problems of management and the need to treat two concurrent illnesses simultaneously.

In addition to this difficulty, the question has been frequently asked whether the existence of the chronic emotional disturbance—with its anxiety, with its feelings of hopelessness and helplessness—may not, in itself, through psycho-endocrine pathways, influence the malignancy and the course of that disease. Some investigators have raised the question whether such emotional crises and disturbances may not contribute to the organic condition by modifying or impairing the immune responses of the patient. There is considerable evidence to suggest that individuals who develop cancer have had their immune responses impaired by certain factors including illness (both organic and emotional), chemical agents, or virus (Weksler, 1973). Dr. Jack Katz et al., in the Second Conference of Psychophysiological Aspects of Cancer 1969), raises the question whether "breast cancer exacerbation during periods of emotional crisis may be mediated via such psychoendocrine pathways."

There must be similar attention paid to the emotional disturbance developing subsequent to an organic condition, because of the possibility that it may worsen or aggravate the original organic condition. Reference is being made here to the anxiety and depression that are anticipated as normal and reasonable responses to the loss of a breast in the woman and to the knowledge that she has cancer. Since it was always felt that such emotional reactions were appropriate and "normal," they have been, more or less, ignored. Many surgeons wisely warn their patients that following mastectomy there will inevitably be feelings of depression and worry, but that they are to be considered usual and normal and that, it is hoped, they will subside and eventually disappear. This may occur in many instances, but in a significant percentage of women the reaction is severe and prolonged.

Recent findings and discussions suggest that such emotional responses may produce physiological concomitants which, through autonomic and neuro-endocrine pathways, may cause secondary enzymatic and hormonal changes. There is some evidence to suggest that such stress may stimulate adrenal-cortical steriod hormones, which may be immunosuppressive (Solomon, 1969).

The suggestion has been made that increasing levels of catecholamines and glucocorticoids may exercise a destructive effect on the underlying organic condition. It is quite possible that such physiological responses to emotional disturbance, even when the emotional response is temporary, can suppress or modify immune systems enough to influence the growth or spread of neoplastic cells.

This is not considered to be a specific effect on malignancy. For instance, it is generally accepted that suppression of immune systems by various factors, including age, illness, chemicals, etc. can permit invasion and growth of bacterial agents, resulting in infection and clinical illness. Similarly, there has been considerable evidence to suggest that the emotional disturbance, including anxiety and depression, that frequently follows an acute myocardial infarction, can cause elevation of corticosteriod levels which may result in hypoxia of heart muscle and disturbed cardiac function, putting the patient at risk for a possible fatal arrhythmia.

This area of interaction of diseases, where one illness influences the other, still requires much investigation and study, but there have been suggestions, based on some evidence, that when the coping mechanisms of the woman with malignant disease are low, when her defenses are depleted or ineffective, there results a poor prognosis, perhaps because of elevated corticosteroid levels. And under these circumstances, breast cancer exacerbations may occur during emotional disturbances (Katz et al., 1969).

It has been reported that women who reacted to their organic condition and surgery with feelings of fright and despair were more apt to have elevated corticosteroid rates of production (Katz et al., 1969). Those women who presented "giving up" attitudes, with hopelessness and helplessness, showed similar elevations of catecholamines. This must be seen and understood only as a permissive or facilitating factor in the growth or spread of neoplastic cells through endocrine immunological mechanisms. The facilitating effect of such immunological impairment may, of course, influence other diseases.

All of these new suggestions, based on increasing knowledge, should make us think that the so-called normal and understandable emotional responses to cancer and to mastectomy in our patients may not be as innocuous as has heretofore been accepted. These feelings may have to be regarded as potentially dangerous and therefore such emotional reactions, acute or chronic, should be actively and aggressively treated whenever they are recognized. To ignore such symptoms, on the basis that they are appropriate or usual, may encourage us to neglect one pathway that can contribute a significant destructive influence on the underlying disease and its progression.

Conclusion

The purpose of the above brief comments has been to emphasize some of the psychological aspects of mastectomy. Recommendations have been made which, it is believed, could reduce psychiatric sequelae and complications of loss of a breast. It is felt that awareness of these factors and of the emotional needs of women exposed to this trauma will further good patient care, which will, in turn, improve and enhance these women's subsequent lives.

REFERENCES

Ervin, C.V., Jr. Psychological Adjustment to Mastectomy. *Medical Aspects of Human Sexuality.* 7:11, 1973.

Harrell, H.C. To lose a breast. *Amer. J. Nursing,* :676, 1972.

Katz, J. et al. Psychoendocrine consideration in cancer of the breast. Second Conference on Psychophysiological Aspects of Cancer. *Annal of The New York Acad. Sciences.* 164:509, 1969.

Markel, W.M. The American Cancer Society's program for the rehabilitation of the breast cancer patient. *Cancer,* 28:1676, 1971.

Solomon, G.F. Emotion, stress, the central nervous system and immunity. Second Conference on Psychophysiological Aspects of Cancer. *Annals of the New York Acad. Sciences.* 164:335, 1969.

Weksler, M.E. Immunology & Cancer. *New York State J. Med.* 73:544, 1973.

Zalan, J. *I Am Whole Again.* New York: Random House, 1978 p.127.

CHAPTER 6

Use of Nuclear Medicine In The Management Of Patients With Cancer Of The Breast

ABRAHAM GEFFEN

SKELETAL SCREENING FOR OCCULT METASTASES IN PRIMARY BREAST CANCER

Bone is often the first site of metastatic or recurrent disease in breast cancer. Considerable interest has been directed to determine the value of bone scanning with radioactive pharmaceuticals (radionuclides) for early detection of metastatic or recurrent breast cancer. Charkes et al. (1968) reported success in detecting skeletal metastases from various primary sites with the use of the radioactive strontium bone scan. Radioactive fluorine-18 has also been successfully used for bone scanning (Galasko et al., 1968; Galasko 1972). The advent of a new generation of bone scanning agents, namely, technetium-99m-labeled polyphosphate and its analogues, has greatly improved the results.

Weber et al. (1974) have documented the value of technetium-99m-labeled polyphosphate and its analogues in comparison with flourine-18. The technetium-99m-labeled polyphosphates are readily made from generator-produced technetium-99m pertechnate, which is widely available.

The rationale for the localization of radionuclides in the bones has been summarized very adequately (O'Mara and Charkes, 1975). Strontium-85 is injected intravenously as chloride or nitrate, 100 microcuries per dose. The radionuclide exchanges with stable strontium and substitutes for calcium ions (heterionic transfer) in amorphous calcium phosphate and on the surface of the hydroxyapatite crystal lattice of newly formed osteoid. Fluorine-18 is injected as sodium fluoride, one to four millicuries per dose. The fluoride ions exchange for the hydroxyl group in hydroxyapatite on the surface of the bone crystal, then pass into the interior of the crystal by heterionic exchange.

Technetium-99m is injected as a complex with either polyphosphate, pyrophosphate, or diphosphonate. The complexes are believed to be absorbed on the surface of the bone crystals. In normal bone the radionuclides are deposited primarily in the areas of new bone formation, such as, in the calcifying cartilage of the metaphyses, in the cortex where periosteal and endosteal appositional growth occurs, and in the trabecular bone. The tracer is taken up in the amorphous calcium phosphate and hydroxyapatite crystals in the newly deposited immature osteoid. As mineralization proceeds, the rate of tracer uptake reaches a peak and then diminishes, so that fully calcified bone takes up relatively little of the radionuclide. Uptake of the radioactive tracer is also affected by alterations in blood flow, temperature, hormonal influences, and renal clearance. Thus, the pertechnate complexes may present many normal areas of activity in the skeleton, so that one must learn to recognize normal bone scans in order to diagnose abnormalities.

The pathophysiology of abnormal bone scans rests mainly on the fact that bone usually reacts to the presence of metastatic cancer by forming new bone ("reactive bone"). This new bone begins as immature osteoid tissue, which is laid down by proliferating osteoblasts. In this matrix, hydroxyapatite crystals form, and it is the interaction of tracers with these crystals that forms the basis of bone scanning (Charkes, W.D., 1972). Much of the basic study has been performed with strontium-85 (Charkes et al., 1968). The exact mechanisms of uptake of the technetium-99m-labeled complexes have not fully been worked out, but are assumed to be similar.

There is no reaction of the patient to these radionuclides. They do cross the placental barrier. Strontium-85 is contraindicated in pregnancy. Low doses of fluorine-18 and technetium-99m may be safe near term. We know that 10% of injected strontium-85 appears in milk. Therefore, bone scans with strontium-85 are contraindicated in nursing women.

Bone scintiscans with technetium-99m polyphosphates are obtained with a rectilinear scanner, preferably dual probe, in a 5:1 minification mode. They can also be obtained with gamma camera scintiphotography. The dose of technetium-99m-labeled polyphosphate is usually 12 to 15 millicuries. Bone scintiscans are obtained four hours after injection of the tracer. The patient receives copious amounts of fluid orally to minimize bladder visualization. Anterior and posterior views of the skeleton, with lateral views of the skull, are obtained. With the gamma camera technique, the hands and feet may not be routinely visualized. Lentle et al. (1975) report an acceptable radiation level of approximately 450 millirads from a 15 millicurie dose of technetium-99m-labeled polyphosphate and its analogues.

Galasko (1972), in studying 127 women with advanced breast cancer, included careful clinical examination, x-ray skeletal surveys, and blood chemistries. The last 50 of this group of 127 women also had skeletal scintigrams with 1.5 millicuries of fluorine-18; 86 of the 127 developed x-ray evidence of skeletal metastases and 25 of the last 50 (who had the radionuclide bone scans) had x-ray evidence of skeletal metastases, as compared with 42 (84%) who had positive scintigrams—and in 36 of these there were more lesions seen on the radionuclide scan than on x-ray. All of the 42 women with positive scintigrams had their cancers confirmed clinically within 18 months.

Of more interest to this discussion, intended to elucidate the detection of occult metastases, the same author studied another group of 50 patients having breast cancer, with *no* clinical evidence of metastases and with *negative* skeletal x-rays, using the same radionuclide. The author designated this second group of 50 women as "early" breast cancer. The scan was positive in 12 (24%) patients, the metastases confirmed clinically in 10 of the 12 women by the end of 30 months. Five (13%) of the 38 negative scans developed metastases or local recurrence within 30 months.

On a third group, 18 patients were thought to have breast cancer (but whose lesions proved to be benign histologically), radionuclide scans (18-fluoride) were performed. This group, designated by the same author as "controls," all had normal scans. Galasko concluded that the radionuclide scan (fluorine-18) was more accurate and more sensitive for early detection of skeletal metastases from breast cancer than was the x-ray skeletal survey.

In a study designed to attempt to demonstrate the presence of bone metastases in women being evaluated for the presence of cancer of the breast prior to undergoing definitive surgical treatment, Opler (1974) reported on a preliminary series. He utilized the newer bone imaging radionuclides, technetium-99m-labeled diphosphonates, with gamma camera scanning technique; 14% of the patients showed changes consistent with metastases. The follow-up later documented that the disease had indeed spread in 14% of these women prior to surgery. Opler concluded that the radionuclide bone scan should result in a more accurate method of staging breast cancer and should aid in selecting rational forms of treatment for the patient with disseminated breast cancer.

Although differing in detection rates (14% and 24%) in finding occult metastatic breast cancer, these two studies both provided valid positive results for encouraging others to accumulate more data. The difference in the specific percentages detected by the radionuclide bone scans in the two studies may be the result of differences in population or patient selection.

Citrin et al. (1975), using technetium-99m phosphate, studied 190 patients with breast cancer, comparing the radionuclide bone scan and the x-ray skeletal survey; 70 control subjects were also included. The patients were not graded or grouped into clinical stages, but were divided into three study groups:

1) 47 patients with known bony metastases (x-ray positive) who were scanned to permit development and validation of the technique.

2) 60 patients in whom there was a clinical suspicion of metastases but no definite lesion seen on x-rays.

3) 83 patients scanned at the time of initial and primary treatment.

Of the 47 patients in the first group (all with positive x-rays), the scintiscan was positive in all but two. The latter two patients had known bony metastases for five years with sclerosis of the sites that were negative on bone scan and, therefore, the metastases were considered to be inactive. However, in 24 (50%) patients the scan showed more lesions than had been seen on x-ray.

In the second group (clinical suspicion of metastases, but negative x-rays), the scan was positive in 28 (48%) patients. In the third group (negative x-ray survey and no clinical suspicion of bone metastases), 24 (27%) women had positive scintiscans, suggesting occult metastases. In the control group (70 patients), there were two false positives.

Lentle et al. (1975) studied 174 unselected patients with cancer of the breast (consecutive and previously untreated patients "newly diagnosed"), staged according to the International Cancer TNM classification. X-ray skeletal surveys and radionuclide bone scans were obtained either prior to biopsy or operation or immediately after operation. (Bone scans were done with a dual probe rectilinear scanner, supplemented when necessary with gamma camera scinitiphotographs.) Technetium-99m-polyphosphate (12 to 14 millcuries) was the radionuclide used. Nine of the patients had both scintiscan and x-ray evidence of metastatic disease involving bone. In nine other patients, the scintiscan was positive and the x-ray survey was negative. Five of the latter developed x-ray evidence of metastases at precisely the sites anticipated by the abnormal bone scan. In 10 patients with normal bone scans at the time of initial diagnosis, there was evidence by scintiscan of bone metastases on follow-up study; eight of these patients developed metastases within a year.

The authors conclude that their data suggest that the bone scan permits the diagnosis of bone metastases from cancer of the breast in 18 (or 10.3%) of a possible 26 (or 14.9%) of patients in a series of 174. Fifteen patients had other causes for an abnormal bone scan (Paget's disease, osteoarthroses, fibrous dysplasia, fractures, or other trauma). After approrpiate x-ray correlation, such coincidental findings were recognized, and the scintiscans interpreted as negative for metastatic disease. This is a very important aspect of scan interpretation. The authors of this study concluded 1) that bone scanning yields twice the number of positive findings that x-ray surveys yield; 2) that pretreatment bone scans are indicated in patients with newly diagnosed cancer of the breast, Stages III and IV; and 3) that there is an advantage in having a baseline bone scan for evaluating subsequent adverse changes.

Roberts et al. (1976) compared radiography and radionuclide scintigraphy for detecting skeletal metastases in breast cancer. Of 114 patients who had x-rays to detect skeletal metastases, two had positive findings. Bone scans with technetium-99m-labeled polyphosphate or diphosphonate were performed on 46 patients who had negative x-rays for metastases; 11 of the 46 (23%) had positive scans suggestive of metastases (after exclusion of eight "benign" lesions that produced positive scans). The investigators concluded that the radionuclide scan should be used in place of the x-ray bone survey as the initial screening procedure and followed with x-ray study of specific skeletal areas seen as abnormal on the scintiscan.

Citrin et al. (1976) published the results of a prospective study designed to determine the value of the technetium-99m-labeled phosphate bone scan in the preoperative assessment and postoperative follow-up of patients with primary cancer of the breast. They reported on 75 patients, 49 having Stage I cancer and 26 Stage II (International Classification), with a follow-up of up to 34 months.

The initial x-ray survey showed all 75 women to be normal. The bone scan showed 64 to be normal and 11 abnormal initially. The follow-up period has been three to 34 months, with a mean of 16 months. Abnormal bone scans developed in an additional 13 patients, giving a total of 24 abnormal scans. Nine of the 24 women with abnormal bone scans have died; only one of the 51 with normal scans has died, from pulmonary embolus. Five of the women in the normal scan group are alive with no disease in the bone. Of the 15 living women with abnormal bone scans, one has bone metastases, five have recurrent disease other than bone, and nine are without evidence of disease.

The authors conclude "that it is reasonable to treat all patients with abnormal scans with systemic therapy, irrespective of whether or not they have symptoms or x-ray evidence of disease. They also state "that the high incidence of abnormal bone scans in patients with Stage II cancer of the breast makes it clear that the planning of further studies concerning the value of adjuvant chemotherapy, particularly in Stage II cancer, should take the result of the bone scan into consideration".

Campbell et al. (1976) also reported on the value of preliminary bone scanning in staging and assessing the prognosis of breast cancer. They used technetium-99m pyrophosphate with gamma camera imaging. They studied 80 patients with breast cancer. Positive scans due to benign skeletal conditions were identified by x-ray and excluded from the true positive group. The authors found 35% of the patients to be positive, in Stages I and II. The follow-up scans at 12 months showed 54.2% of the original positive scans had evidence of disseminated disease, compared with 5.7% of patients with originally negative scans. At 18 months, 85.7% of the originally positive scan patients had evidence of disseminated disease, compared with 11.4% of the patients with originally negative scans.

The authors concluded that the lesions shown by scanning actually represent metastatic foci and thus determine prognosis. "Scan lesions develop into clinical lesions," they stated. They felt that positive bone scans indicate a need for systemic therapy, and they have planned a prospective clinical trial of adjuvant quadruple chemotherapy for scan-positive and histologically proven Stage II cancer of the breast.

Gerber et al. (1977), using technetium-99m-labeled distannous diphosphate complex, studied 122 patients. They divided them into three groups: Group one, "disease confined to the breast, corresponded to clinical Stage I." Group two, "disease involving breast and regional lymph nodes, corresponded to Stage II." Group three, "preoperative evidence of dissemination, invasion of chest wall, or matting of axillary nodes, corresponded to Stages III and IV." Seven patients (6%) had evidence of bone metastases initially—two of the five patients in Group one and five of the seven in Group three. Of 55 patients with normal preoperative scans, 20 (30%) developed metastases on follow-up scans.

The authors concluded that 1) pre-operative bone scanning will uncover a small number of occult metastases; 2) there is a high scan conversion rate of Stages I and II; therefore, routine periodic bone scans should be obtained ("scan conversion designates the appearance of scan abnormalities suggesting metastases in a patient with a previously normal bone scan"); and 3) it is important to establish a baseline to detect early new scan abnormalities.

Baker et al. (1977) evaluated the use of bone scans as a screening procedure for occult metastases in primary breast cancer. The series consisted of 104 patients who had technetium-99m-phosphate scans prior to mastectomy. Whole body images were obtained with a dual probe rectilinear scanner. In addition, gamma camera images of the entire spine were obtained, as were images of other areas that were equivocally abnormal on the rectilinear scan. The bone scans were classified as "normal" or as demonstrating "areas of increased activity." Those demonstrating areas of increased activity were then classified as "positive" or "negative for metastases" by correlating the bone scan findings with appropriate x-rays. The x-rays were read as 1) "normal," 2) "diagnostic of benign disease" such as degenerative joint disease, trauma, or Paget's disease of the bone, and 3) "diagnostic of metastatic breast cancer."

An abnormal bone scan associated with an area of x-ray normality or with x-ray evidence of metastases was considered positive for metastases. A bone scan showing increased activity associated with a benign x-ray abnormality (e.g., Paget's disease of the bone, degenerative joint disease) was considered negative for metastases. All patients were clinically staged according to the TNM classification system—Stage I ($T_1N_0M_0$), Stage II ($T_1N_1M_0$) or ($T_2N_1M_0$), and Stage III (T_3 or T_4N_0 or N_1M_0). Of the 27 patients in Stage I, only one had an abnormal preoperative bone scan that was confirmed on the x-ray. Eight patients had bone scans classified as normal. The other 18 patients had abnormal bone scans. But all 18 patients had x-ray evidence of either degenerative joint disease or trauma.

Of the 36 Stage II patients, 13 had normal scans, and 23 had abnormal scans, all accounted for by x-ray evidence of benign disease (Paget's disease in one patient and degenerative joint disease in 22). In the 41 Stage III patients, 10 (24%) had positive scans. Two of the 10 had abnormal x-rays also; eight had normal x-rays. Later, in all but one of the eight, metastatic lesions became apparent on x-ray after 16-36 months of follow-up. This demonstrated the increased sensitivity of the radionuclide bone scan compared with that of the x-ray.

These authors concluded that pre-operative bone scans in patients with Stage I and Stage II breast cancer will not reveal a significant number of occult osseous metastases. The value of preoperative bone scans in Stages I and II is to provide a baseline for comparison with subsequent scans obtained. The authors do recommend routine preoperative bone scanning in the preoperative assessment of Stage III breast cancer patients.

Schaffer et al. (1977) also studied the incidence of bone metastases in women with minimal or occult breast cancer. They defined minimal as less than 5mm and occult as 5mm to 30mm. In 14 patients with minimal breast cancer, bone scans and x-ray skeletal surveys were normal. In the 28 occult group, five women of 28 (18%) had abnormal bone scans and abnormal skeletal surveys. (These five patients had metastatic bone disease; the occult breast cancer was found as a result of the search for an occult primary neoplasm). The conclusions of the authors were similar to those of Baker et al. (1977).

The most recent report (Hammond et al., 1978) is a study of 43 patients who had technetium-99m-labeled pyrophosphate bone scans within two months of mastectomy for breast cancer (Stage I, one patient, Stage II, 28, and Stage III, 14). The initial bone scans were equivocal for six patients and definitely abnormal for six others.

X-rays confirmed metastases in two patients who were then excluded from the series. Of the 41 remaining, serial bone scans were unchanged in 20 patients who had no clinical recurrence after 20 months of follow-up.

Clinical recurrence occurred in six of 16 patients whose serial bone scans showed either appearance of new focal lesions or disappearance of old lesions (at 43 months follow-up).

The authors concluded that 1) initial and serial bone scanning are important aspects in the development of a rational adjuvant therapy program; 2) bone scans should be performed prior to adjuvant treatment to detect overt metastatic disease; and 3) the use of serial bone scans should enable one to select a subgroup of patients with a high risk of recurrence who might benefit from more intensive or more prolonged adjuvant therapy in an effort to reduce their risk of subsequent recurrence.

Similar conclusions by Citrin et al. (1977), based on their own studies and those of others quoted above, were suggested: "The short-term prognosis for scan-positive patients is poor. Serial bone scans provide a safe and reliable prognostic index in patients following mastectomy. The bone scan can be developed as one component of a matrix of diagnostic tests designed to provide prognostic information leading to earlier and more rational therapeutic programs in individual patients."

Conclusions and Recommendations

1) Routine preoperative bone radionuclide scanning is not an effective means for detecting occult metastases in clinical Stages I and II breast cancer. There is an advantage, however, in having a baseline scan to detect early new scan abnormalities.

2) Routine periodic postmastectomy bone scanning in clinical Stages I and II may be of value because of the high potential of occult spread already present with the subsequent appearance of scan abnormalities in a patient with a previously normal bone scan. It is probably advisable to perform bone scans at six-month intervals after mastectomy for the first two to three years, annually the fourth and fifth years, then as warranted by symptoms.

3) Routine preoperative bone scan should be obtained in all patients with clinical Stage III cancer.

4) Pre-operative bone scanning should replace the x-ray survey.

5) Skeletal x-rays may be used to confirm or assess localized areas detected on the radionuclide scan.

6) An abnormal bone scan with a negative x-ray is presumptive evidence for metastases.

BONE SCANS IN STAGE IV BREAST CANCER

Prior to the introduction of the bone seeking radionuclides, x-rays of the skeleton were the primary method of documenting symptomatic and occult bony metastases in clinical Stage IV breast cancer. As quoted above (Citrin et al., 1975), it has been shown that in 47 patients with both positive x-rays and positive radionuclide scans more lesions were demonstrated on the scintiscan (24, or 50%) than on the x-rays. Similar findings were reported by Galasko (1972) and Galasko et al., (1972). It appears, therfore, that serial bone scans rather than frequent skeletal x-ray surveys will provide an earlier index of the progression of metastatic disease. This does not preclude the use of x-rays of the skeleton to focus on the areas localized on the bone scan and to demonstrate such lesions with more definitive and comprehensive anatomical details.

Sklaroff et al. (1976) have listed other indications for bone scanning for patients with bone metastases from breast cancer. They suggest its use to examine patients with persistent pain thought to be in the bone despite equivocal or negative x-rays, to evaluate areas that are difficult to study by conventional x-ray methods, such as the sternum and scapula, to differentiate pathologic from traumatic fracture by demonstrating other sites of involvement not apparent on x-rays, to plan radiation therapy portals, and to determine the response to hormonal, chemical, or radiation therapy. The latter value of bone scanning has been advanced also by Galasko et al. (1972A) and Citrin et al. (1974). These authors feel that serial bone scans can provide a quantitative method of assessing the response to various therapeutic regimes and that this use of bone scanning may well represent the most important therapeutic application of bone scanning in breast cancer.

Recommendations

1) Skeletal radionuclide scans should be taken before the start of therapy (radiation, chemical, or hormonal).

2) Skeletal x-rays of all areas positive on radionuclide bone scan are recommended.

3) Periodic (three-to six-month intervals) skeletal scans should be taken to evaluate response to therapy.

4) Parallel serial x-rays of the specific abnormal areas localized on the scan are advised at more frequent intervals if necessary, with special attention to pathological fractures in critical locations that may necessitate urgent or emergent supportive surgical or orthopedic intervention.

RADIONUCLIDE LIVER SCANS IN CANCER OF THE BREAST

Preoperative (Clinical Stages I, II, and III) screening for occult liver metastases

The current agent of choice for static examination of the liver is sulfur colloid labeled with technetium-99m. The rationale and the technique for the use of this nuclide have been summarized by Johnson (1975) and by Shingleton (1972). The adult dose is 1 to 3 millcuries. The scintillation camera is preferable, although the rectilinear scanner may also be used.

Imaging is begun five minutes after injection. Anterior, posterior, and lateral scans are obtained. Normal areas concentrate the radioactive nuclide, which is taken up by the Kupffer cells of the reticulo-endothelial system (not by the polygonal hepatic cells). Masses that replace or displace the normal hepatic tissue appear as areas of decreased density (cold areas).

The most widely used indication for liver scanning is suspected metastatic tumors. A metastatic lesion less than 2.0 cm in size is too small to be detected by present scanning methods. A 4 cm lesion may well be undetected if situated centrally in the right lobe. Despite the limitations of the liver scan, there have been significant studies evaluating the place of the liver scan and of liver function tests in the diagnosis of occult liver metastases.

Wiener and Sachs (1978), in a retrospective review of 234 patients, reported that the liver scan detected only one patient with unsuspected metastases. There were eight false-positive studies. Abnormal liver chemistry tests identified liver metastases in an additional 19 patients in a follow-up group of 192 patients. The results confirmed previous studies (Sears et al., 1975) showing a low yield for liver scan in the diagnosis of unsuspected liver metastases.

Pitfalls in detection by and interpretation of liver scans have been emphasized (Covington, 1970). False positives in both the initial and follow-up scans are significant, 12% to 62%, as are false negatives, ranging from 5% to 25% (Oxley, 1975; Galasko, 1975). There are limitations of the liver scan because of limited resolution of the equipment, depth of lesions, and motion (Castagna et al., 1972). There is also inherent difficulty of detection which is related to the characteristic pattern of involvement (Rosenthal et al., 1973). The false positives may be due to many conditions, such as, unusual variants, inflammatory disease, and benign neoplasms (Oxley, 1975; Galasko 1975).

The combined use of liver function tests and liver scans has been advocated (Castagna et al. 1972). Wiener et al. (1978) concluded that liver chemistries separated true from false positive scans for both the initial and follow-up groups, and that the liver function tests are of little help in the presence of normal scans. Rosenthal et al. (1973) and Wiener et al. (1978) have suggested that because of the low yield of detection of hepatic metastases in the initial work-up of breast cancer patients, routine liver function tests should be abandoned unless there is evidence of abnormal liver function. Krutchik et al. (1978) took issue with Wiener and Sachs, stating 1) that liver function tests are not reliable, citing elevation of alkaline phosphatase 10% to 80% above normal when no metastases were present (Ferrier et al., 1969); and 2) that metastatic disease to the liver may have normal alkaline phosphatase in 20% to 50% of cases (Almersjö et al., 1974).

Other studies have also questioned the accuracy of the liver function tests. Baum et al. (1966) and Gollin et al. (1964) stated that there is a higher incidence of false results with serum alkaline phosphatase determinations than with scintillation imaging. Jhingran et al. (1971) noted a false positive rate of 41% with the alkaline phosphatase level, compared with a 9% rate with imaging. Watson et al. (1970) reported normal liver function tests in 19 of 36 patients with proven metastases to the liver. Wilson et al. (1969) pointed out that when both the scintiscan and the alkaline phosphatase levels are normal, the likelihood of focal disease is remote. They found that only one of 23 patients with combined negative results had metastases to the liver.

Although combined use of liver function tests and liver scans may reduce the number of false positives, the limitations of the liver scan preclude its routine use for the detection of occult metastases in breast cancer Stages I, II, and III.

Liver Scan in Clinical Stage IV

In Stage IV cancer of the breast, liver scanning is of value as a non-invasive technique to document and localize hepatic metastases. The status of hepatic metastases and their response to therapy (radiation, hormonal, or chemotherapy) can be effectively and objectively determined by serial liver scan examinations (Hanson et al., 1963).

RADIONUCLIDE BRAIN SCANNING IN CLINICAL STAGE IV BREAST CANCER

The current agent of choice for static brain scanning is technetium-99m pertechnate. The mechanism of localization in abnormal lesions in the brain is not completely understood. There is "a disturbance in the blood-brain barrier," as a result of the action of brain capillaries passing sub-stances into the extra-cellular spaces and very selective free transport of specific narrow classes of substances (Schall et al., 1972).

The technetium-99m pertechnate brain scan is not useful as a screening test in finding small occult lesions. However, it is of significant value as a non-invasive technique for documentation and localization of metastatic le-sions in the brain. The brain scan is also of value as a periodic follow-up ex-amination to assess the effectiveness of therapy (radiation, hormonal, steroids, or chemotherapy) (Holmes et al., 1975).

NEWER SCANNING TECHNIQUES

Computerized Axial Tomography

This method (abbreviated CAT or CT) is the most exciting and revolu-tionary radiological diagnostic advance since the actual discovery of x-rays (Hounsfield et al., 1973). The full effect of this technique has not as yet been realized. It may be applied to all areas of the human body—the head, tho-rax, breasts, abdomen, pelvis, or extremities. Images of cross-sectional or axial slices of predetermined thickness of the anatomical area selected may be obtained with accuracy to the millimeter. This method opens up new vis-tas for screening for occult cancer.

Computerized Positron Emission Tomography

This technique applies the principles of CAT scanning to nuclear emis-sion sources rather than x-ray sources, and is also a revolutionary advance in nuclear scanning. The development of this methodology may lower the threshold of detectability in liver scanning to the range of 1.0 cm to 2.0 cm (Johnson, 1975).

Ultrasonography

This modality has already been used in liver scanning. The ultrasound scan is less sensitive in detecting a localized intrahepatic abnormality than the radionuclide scan but yields a lower rate of false positive diagnoses of diffuse hepatic disease. Johnson (1975) indicates that the present evidence suggests that the combined results of the radionuclide liver scan and the ul-trasound scan "may be more accurate than those of either method individually. The noninvasiveness of ultrasound and its lack of morbidity and absence of ionizing radiation commend its use."

REFERENCES

Almersjö, O., Bengmark, S., Hafström, L., Rosengren, K. A comparative study using serum tests, angiography, scintiscanning, and laparotomy. *Am. J. Surg.* 27:663, 1974.

Baker, E.R., Holmes, E.R., Alderson, O.O., Khouri, N.F., Wagner, H.N. An evaluation of bone scans as screening procedures for occult metastases in primary breast cancer. *Annals Surg.* 186:363, 1977.

Baum, S., Silver, L., Vouchides, D. Recognition of hepatic metastases through radioisotope color scanning *J.A.M.A.* 197:675, 1966.

Campbell, D.J., Banks, A.J., Oates, G.D. Value of preliminary bone scanning in staging and assessing the prognosis of breast cancer. *Br. J. Surg.* 63:811, 1976.

Castagna, J., Benfield, J.R., Yamada, H., Johnson, D.E. The reliability of liver scans and function tests in detecting metastases. *Surg. Gyn. & Obs.* 134:463, 1972.

Charkes, N.D., Young, J., Sklaroff, D.M. The pathological basis of the strontium bone scan. *J.A.M.A.* 206:2482, 1968.

Charkes, N.D. In *Nuclear Medicine.* Blahd, W.H. (ed.), New York: McGraw-Hill, 1972, pp. 470-477.

Citrin, D.L., Bessent, R.G., Tuohy, J.B., Grieg, W.R., Blumgart, L.H. Quantitative bone scanning: a method for assessing response of bone metastases to treatment. *Lancet* 1:1132, 1974.

Citrin, D.L., Bessent, R.G., Grieg, W.R., McKellar, N.J., Furnival, C., Blumgart, L.H. The application of the 99Tc^mphosphate bone scan to the study of breast cancer. *Br. J. Surg.* 62:201, 1975.

Citrin, D.L., Furnival, C.M., Bessent, R.G., Grieg, W.R., Bell, G., Blumgart, L.H. Radioactive technetium phosphate bone scanning in preoperative assessment and follow-up study of patients with primary cancer of the breast. *Surg. Gyn. & Obs.* 143:360, 1976

Citrin, D.L., Tormey, D.C., Carbone, P.P. Implications of the 99mtechnetium diphosphonate bone scan on treatment of primary breast cancer. *Canc. Treatment Reports* 61:1249, 1977.

Covington, E.E. Pitfalls in liver photoscan. *Am.J. Roentg.* 109:745, 1970.

Ferrier, F.L., Hatcher, C.R., Achord, J.L. The value of liver scanning for detection of metastatic cancer. *Am. Sug.* 35:112, 1969.

Galasko, C.S.B., Westerman, B., Li, J., Sellwood, R.A., Burn, J.I. Use of gamma camera for early detection of osseous metastases from mammary cancer. *Br. J. Surg.* 55:613, 1968.

Galasko, C.S.B. Skeletal metastases and mammary cancer. *Ann. R. Coll. Surg. Engl.* 50:3, 1972.

Galasko, C.S.B., Doyle, F.H. The detection of skeletal metastases from mammary cancer; a regional comparison between radiology and scintigraphy. *Clin. Rad.* 23:295, 1972.

Galasko, C.S.B., Doyle, F.H. The response to therapy of skeletal metastases from mammary cancer: assessment by scintigraphy. *Br. J. Surg.* 59:85, 1972A.

Galasko, C.S.B. The value of scintigraphy in malignant disease. *Cancer Treat. Rev.* 2:225, 1975.

Gerber, F.H., Goodreau, J.J. Kirschner, P.T., Fouty, W.J. Efficacy of preoperative and postoperative bone scanning in the management of breast cancer. *New Eng. J. Med.* 297:300, 1977.

Gollin, F.F., Sims, J.L. Cameron, J.R. Liver scanning and liver function tests. J.A.M.A. 187:111, 1964.

Hammond, N., Jones, S.E., Salmon, S.E., Patton, D., Woolfenden, J. Predictive value of bone scans in an adjuvant breast cancer program. *Cancer* 41:138, 1978.

Hanson, D.J., Soule, A.B., Peterson, O.S., Haines, C.R., Janney, C.D. Liver photoscanning in evaluation of cancer chemotherapy. *Arch. Surg.* 87:442, 1963.

Holmes, R.A. and Staab, E.V. in Freeman, L.M. Johnson, P.M. Clinical Scintillation Imaging. In *The Central Nervous System.* New York: Grune & Stratton, 1975, pp. 247-323.

Hounsfield, G.N., Ambrose, J. Computerized transverse axial scanning (tomography) *Br. J. Rad.* 46:1016, 1973.

Jhingran, S.G., Jorda, L., Jahus, M.F., Haynie, T.P. Liver scintigrams compared with alkaline phosphatase and BSP determinations in the detection of metastatic carcinoma. *J. Nucl. Med.* 12:227, 1971.

Johnson, P.M. In Freeman, L.M. and Johnson, P.M. *Clinical Scintillation Imaging.* New York: Grune & Stratton, 1975, pp. 405-459.

Krutchik, A.N., Buzdor, A.V. Letter to editor. *Arch. Surg.* 113:1110, 1978.

Lentle, B.C., Burns, P.E., Dierich, H., Jackson, F.I. Bone scintiscanning in the initial assessment of carcinoma of the breast. *Surg. Gyn. & Obs.* 141:43, 1975.

O'Mara, R.E., Charkes, N.D. In *Clinical Scintillation Imaging.* Freeman, L.W., Johnson, P.M. (eds.). New York: Grune & Stratton, 1975, pp. 555-565.

Opler, S.R. Bone scanning in staging breast cancer. *Proc Am. Assoc. Cancer Res.* 15:47, 1974.

Oxley, D. Nuclear diagnosis of disseminated cancer of the breast. *Am. J. Clin. Path.* 64:780, 1975.

Roberts, J.G., Bligh, A.S., Gravelle, I.H., Leach, K.G., Baum, M. Evaluation of radiography and isotopic scintigraphy for detecting skeletal metastases in breast cancer. *Lancet* 1:237, 1976.

Rosenthal, S., Kaufman, S. The liver scan in metastatic disease. *Arch. Surg.* 106:656, 1973.

Schaffer, D.L., Kalisher, L. Incidence of bone metastases in women with minimal and occult breast carcinoma. *Radiology* 124:675, 1977.

Schall, G.L. Quinn, J.L.III In *Nuclear Medicine.* Blahd, W.H., (ed.). New York: McGraw-Hill, 1972, pp. 238-240, 259-260.

Sears, H.F., Gerber, F.H., Sturtz, D.L. Liver scan and carcinoma of the breast. *Surg. Gyn. & Obs.* 140:409, 1975.

Shingelton, W.W. In *Nuclear Medicine* Blahd, W.H. (ed.). New York: McGraw-Hill, 1972.

Sklaroff, R.B. Sklaroff, D.M. Bone metastases from breast cancer at the time of radical mastectomy as detected by bone scan. Eight year follow-up. *Cancer* 38:107, 1976.

Watson, A., Torrance, H.B. Liver scanning in surgical practice. *Br. J. Surg.* 405, 1970.

Weber, D.A., Keyes, J.W., Landman, S., Wilson, G.A. Comparison of Technetium 99m polyphosphate and F 18 for bone imaging. *Am. J. Roentg.* 121:184, 1974.

Wiener, S.N., Sachs, S.H. An assessment of routine liver scanning in patients with breast cancer. *Arch. Surg.* 113:126, 1978.

Wilson, F.E., Preston, D.F., Overholt, E.L. Detection of hepatic neoplasm. J.A.M.A. 209:676, 1969.

CHAPTER 7

The Pathologist's Role In The Diagnosis And Treatment Of Breast Cancer

ADA B. CHABON

The outlook for patients with breast cancer has improved. This is clear because the incidence of the disease has increased at the same time that mortality rates have decreased (Cutler et al., 1971). What explains this improvement? There are three possibilities: 1) treatment is better; 2) diagnosis is being established at an earlier stage of the disease; 3) there has been some basic change in the biologic behavior of breast cancer (Black et al., 1972). I know of no concrete evidence that there has been any basic change in the biologic characteristics or behavior of breast cancer. We must therefore look to other factors to explain the observed improvement in breast cancer prognosis.

What about "better treatment" as the explanation? There is no doubt that promising claims have been advanced by surgeons, radiotherapists, and chemotherapists (Bonadonna et al., 1976; Fisher, 1973; Fisher et al., 1975; Lippman et al., 1978; Schottenfeld et al., 1976; Schwartz et al., 1978; Urban, 1977). In particular various combinations of therapy, especially chemotherapy as an adjuvant to surgical intervention, have been proclaimed to lengthen the disease-free interval after primary operation. Yet these results have been viewed with guarded optimism (Culliton, 1976), even by those directly involved in the clinical trials (Bonadonna et al., 1976; Fisher, 1973).

The appearance of hormone receptor testing of breast cancer specimens has helped to distinguish those patients who are likely to respond to hormonal manipulation from those who will not (Horowitz et al., 1977; McGuire et al., 1975; McGuire et al., 1977). This would seem to be particularly applicable to patients whose tumors show receptor-positive activity in relation to both estrogen and progesterone (McGuire et al., 1975; McGuire et al.,

1977). Promising as this may be, there are definite problems related to this approach to evaluating breast tumors. Notably, there is the problem of tissue requirements for valid evaluation. A minimum of 1 gm of tumor tissue, well-stripped of adherent fat, is required for valid hormone receptor testing; but today many tumors are too small to provide so much tissue. To be sure, morphologists do not require such large quantities of tumor tissue, so these structure-oriented enthusiasts are avidly seeking morphologic characteristics that will project with equal accuracy the likelihood of breast tumor response to hormonal manipulation (McDivitt, 1978; Pertschuk et al., 1978; Terenius et al., 1974). To date these aspirations have not been fully achieved (McDivitt, 1978; Terenius et al., 1974).

Let us examine the third possibility, viz., that earlier diagnosis may be an important factor in the recently improved outlook for breast cancer patients. In this connection it is important to clarify what is meant by early diagnosis. The concept of minimal breast cancer was originally introduced by Gallager and Martin (1971) who restricted the term to three clearly distinguishable categories: lobular carcinoma in situ, non-invasive intraductal carcinoma, and invasive carcinoma no larger than 0.5 cm in diameter (Gallager, 1976; Gallager and Martin, 1971). Urban (1977) modified the concept to include patients with infiltrating cancer less than 1.0 cm in diameter, but without clinical evidence of axillary metastasis. Hutter (1971) broadened the term "minimal" to include certain tumors with a generally favorable prognosis, such as medullary carcinoma with lymphocytic infiltration, tubular carcinoma, mucinous carcinoma, noninfiltrating Paget's disease of the nipple, and carcinoma arising in a fibroadenoma. Everyone seems to agree that these lesions, as well as the in situ and minimally invasive carcinomas, have fewer axillary metastases and an overall better long-term prognosis.

How does such early diagnosis come about? Largely, it is due to improved methods of detection (Urban, 1976). With increased awareness of the adult female population, self-examination and screening programs have become popular and undoubtedly contribute to early detection of breast disease (Greenwald et al., 1978). Mammography, however, was a most important development for clinical recognition of early breast carcinoma, even at a prepalpable stage (Egan, 1975; Gallager et al., 1969; Koehl et al., 1970; Urban, 1976). According to one authority (Urban, 1976) mammography detects more than 50% of minimal breast carcinoma. The recent discrimination of different mammographic parenchymal patterns holds out the possibility for an even greater yield of such minute neoplasms (Wolfe, 1976).

The success of mammography has posed significant problems that require close, harmonious working relationships between the surgeon and pathologist. Without this, it is possible that mammographically detected, non-palpable lesions may be left behind or incompletely sampled at the time of surgery (Egan, 1975). Moreover, even when surgical excision is successful, the pathologist is now increasingly confronted with tiny and borderline lesions that tax his diagnostic capabilities. Thus, the pathologist must be able to evaluate subtle changes, such as atypical ductal hyperplasia and atypical papillomatosis, and to distinguish such atypical proliferative lesions from in situ carcinoma as well as from small invasive neoplasms. These interpretations, when adequately communicated to the surgeon, will instigate appropriate patient evaluations for concurrent carcinoma and will initiate follow-up programs for early detection of a subsequent cancer.

The advent of mammography has also placed upon the pathologist the need to be familiar with the radiologic appearances of suspicious breast lesions. In fact, specimen radiography has evolved as a useful technique in the analysis of non-palpable breast lesions (Bauermeister et al., 1973; Egan et al., 1969; Gallager, 1975; Rosen et al., 1974). The following approach can be recommended. First, the radiologist locates the suspicious area on the mammogram. The surgeon removes that area, and this is confirmed by radiography of the intact specimen. The specimen is then sliced in breadloaf manner, with individual sections measuring 1 cm or less in thickness. These sections are arranged in sequence on a clear radiographic film, numbered, and another x-ray is taken. The pathologist can now compare the radiogram of the slices with the intact specimen radiogram, and the appropriate segment(s) can be selected for frozen section.

In general, the frozen section technique permits immediate discrimination between benign and malignant tumors, but occasionally the decision is difficult, as may be the case with the atypical proliferative lesions. At other times, the suspicious area is too small to allow diagnosis based on the frozen section procedure. In such circumstances, the importance of mutual respect between surgeon and pathologist becomes apparent. If the surgeon has confidence in the pathologist's judgment, he will not attempt to force an instantaneous diagnosis. Rather the surgeon will defer definitive therapy while the pathologist assures urgent processing of the biopsy so that a firm diagnosis can be reached within 24 hours or so.

Whether the frozen section procedure is followed or the suspect tissue is expeditiously processed for permenent sections, the underlying value of specimen radiography is self-evident. The surgeon knows that he has removed the suspicious lesion detected by mammography, and the pathologist is confident that he has examined this critical area microscopically (Bauermeister et al., 1973; Rosen et al., 1974).

To a large extent mammography depends upon calcification, which is a common feature of malignant breast neoplasms. According to Koehl et al.

(1970), in a series of 450 patients with malignant breast tumors,* 62% had calcification, and this included 32 patients with lobular carcinoma in situ which, as stated above, is grouped with minimal breast carcinoma. Of course, benign lesions may also develop calcification, but the incidence is lower—23% of 1,034 benign lesions in the study cited (Koehl et al., 1970). By specimen radiography, tissue calcification has been found in association with fibroadenomas, sclerosing adenosis, papillomatosis, duct cell hyperplasia, periductal mastitis, and fat necrosis (Snyder et al., 1971). Thus tissue calcification, while not invariably an index of malignancy, is usually indicative of breast pathology and is particularly prevalent in breast cancer.

Specimen radiography as a diagnostic tool is generally considered to be obligatory in a patient with a suspicious mammogram but without a clinically palpable mass. In one study, five of 14 clinically occult carcinomas would have been left behind if this procedure had not been followed (Bauermeister et al., 1973). Although there are differences of opinion about the general usefulness of specimen radiography (Fisher et al., 1974), several investigators (Gallager, 1975; Rosen et al., 1970) advocate the use of this technique for all large breast specimens, for all breast tissue displaying significant atypia or non-invasive carcinoma, and for all biopsies from the opposite breast of patients with known carcinoma in one breast.

This last indication seems particularly germane in view of the high incidence of carcinoma in the opposite breast of patients with a known primary cancer. Some years ago, Leis et al. (1965) called attention to various studies revealing a 7.5% to 10% incidence of bilateral breast carcinoma. These authors (Leis et al., 1965) also presaged general recognition of a group of patients with a high risk of developing carcinoma in the remaining breast—e.g., very young patients especially with a strong family history, patients with a primary mucinous carcinoma or a primary medullary carcinoma with lymphocytic infiltration, women with multiple invasive tumors in the first removed breast, as well as patients with lobular carcinoma in situ (Fukami et al., 1977; Lagios, 1977; Leis et al., 1965; Rosen et al., 1978; Urban, 1977).

Subsequently, Urban et al. (1977) found that contralateral biopsy at the time of primary surgery detects 12.5% of patients as having carcinoma in the remaining breast, although mostly at the "minimal" stage. And McDevitt (1978) has claimed that in patients with primary in situ breast carcinoma, contralateral biopsy will unveil in situ cancer in as many as 20% of cases. Meanwhile, Egan (1976), using a sensitive mammographic technique, has reported a cancer incidence of 7.5% in the second breast. Recently, at Beth Israel Medical Center, New York, Pressman routinely has been taking a mirror-image biopsy from the contralateral breast at the time of surgery for a primary lesion. This procedure has already detected nine cases of unsuspected contralateral in situ carcinoma and 11 cases of atypical duct cell hyperplasia.

Today, therefore, there is broad support and a scientific basis for the concept of contralateral biopsy at the time of surgery for a primary breast cancer. We are particularly concerned about the very young patients and those with a strong family history, and we concur with the view that biopsy tissue removed from the contralateral breast of a patient with a known primary breast cancer should be evaluated by radiologic techniques as well as by careful pathologic studies (Hutter, 1971; Rosen et al., 1970; Snyder et al., 1971). To be sure, the use of such techniques mandates close cooperation among the radiologist, surgeon, and pathologist since their combined efforts must be effectively integrated for optimal results in the care of patients with breast tumors (Egan, 1975; Egan et al., 1969).

Aspiration biopsy of suspicious breast lesions is another method that has emerged in recent years. In some hands (Horowitz et al., 1977; Zajdela et al., 1975), this approach has been highly successful, and cytologic examination of aspiration specimens has, no doubt, contributed to early diagnosis of breast cancer. True, there is the danger of false positive diagnoses; and, to avoid this danger, one apparently must accept a high level of false negative results (Hajdu et al., 1973). Suffice it to say that aspiration biopsy can hardly be recommended as a replacement for surgical biopsy, particularly when aspirates are scanty (Hajdu et al., 1973). Moreover, the interpretive difficulties inherent in the technique cause us to agree with McDevitt (1978) who has said that aspiration biopsy as a routine procedure can hardly be recommended for most practicing pathologists.

In recent years, electron microscopists have extensively explored both benign and malignant breast tumors (Fisher, 1976; Goldenberg et al., 1969; Murad, 1971; Ozello, 1971; Ozello et al., 1970). Although their efforts have produced excellent descriptions of the ultrastructural features of mammary neoplasms, there have been no claims that fine structure can invariably predict the invasive potential of borderline lesions. To be sure, success along these lines could provide another approach to the detection of minimal breast cancer or even precancerous alterations, yet the truth is that the techniques of electron microscopy remain cumbersome and are still not readily available in all institutions where breast cancers are treated. The same might be said for other more specialized techniques, such as the biological or biochemical approaches to the detection of early neoplasia (Gullino, 1977; Jensen et al., 1976; Ludwig et al., 1973).

In brief, early diagnosis, however achieved, does seem to be an important factor in the recently improved outlook for breast cancer patients. This in itself underscores and accentuates the heavy responsibility of the pathologist in current clinical management of breast neoplasms. It is no longer adequate just to determine whether a tumor is benign or malignant, for the pathologist must now also interpret the biological potential of a lesion (Black et al., 1975). The aggressiveness of each cancer must be interpreted in terms of the nuclear grade of the constituent cells and their capacity to invade vascular channels, as well as the quality of the host response, judged from the character and extent of lymphocytic infiltration around the tumor and adjacent venules and the type of reaction in the regional lymph nodes.

Pathologists must be aware that no single factor can determine the outcome of breast cancer. Rather, their importance relates to an ability to integrate a multiplicity of observations for effective projection of the probable behavior of a breast neoplasm. In addition, pathologists must be familiar with statistical probabilities of more extensive involvement of the same or contralateral breast of a patient, and they must be able to communicate this information to the surgeon so that an optimal therapeutic approach can be recommended to the patient.

In reporting, the pathologist is now obliged to provide detailed information on each case. An example of our reporting format follows: A histological description of the tumor and of the surrounding non-involved breast parenchyma is followed by a summary.

Summary-Breast Carcinoma
Tumor size:
Tumor type:
Nuclear grade:
Lymphocytic infiltration:
Vascular invasion:
Lymph nodes:
Sinus histiocytosis:
Estrogen receptor assay:
Progesterone receptor assay:

Complete, detailed reporting that utilizes a common, established nomenclature (Scarff et al., 1968) will enable accurate assessment of the individual patient and, in time, will allow valid studies of data derived from various institutions and geographic areas.

Similar detailed reports are needed for presumptive preneoplastic disease. Thus, it is not acceptable just to diagnose "fibrocystic disease of the breast." Rather, the individual constituent pathologic changes must be spelled out so that valid conclusions can be drawn from the evaluation of large masses of inter-institutional data. Precise and detailed reporting will enable precise and definitive conclusions to be drawn about the relationship between presumptive preneoplastic changes and ensuing or concurrent cancer (Black et al., 1969; Black et al., 1975; Wellings et al., 1975). This will avoid the uncertainties that now exist about such relationships and will open the door to more enlightened prophylactic treatment. Thus, the pathologist has an important, indeed vital, role in specifying the details of each case. There can be no shirking of this responsibility if the pathologist is to be an effective partner in the team approach to optimal care of breast cancer patients.

REFERENCES

Bauermeister, D.E., Hall, McC. H. Specimen radiography. A mandatory adjunct to mammography. *Am. J. Clin. Path.* 59:782, 1973.

Black, M.M., Barclay, T.H.C., Cutler, S.J., Hankey, B.F., Asire, A.J. Association of atypical characteristics of benign breast lesions with subsequent risk of breast cancer. *Cancer* 29:338, 1972.

Black, M.M., Barclay, T.H.C., Hankey, B.F. Prognosis in breast cancer utilizing histologic characteristics of the primary tumor. *Cancer* 36:2048, 1975.

Black, M.M., Chabon, A.B. *In situ* carcinoma of the breast. In *Pathology Annual.* Sommers, S.C. (ed.). New York: Appleton-Century-Crofts, 1969, pp. 185-210.

Black, M.M., deChabon, A.B. *In situ* carcinoma of the breast. In *Genital and Mammary Pathology Decennial, 1966-1975.* Sommers, S.C. (ed.). New York: Appleton-Century-Crofts, 1975, pp. 435-464.

Bonadonna, G., Brusamolino, E., Valagussa, P., Rossi, A., Brugnatelli, L., Brambilla, C., De-Lena, M., Tancini, G., Bajetta, E., Musumeci, R., Veronesi, U. Combination chemotherapy as an adjuvant treatment in operable breast cancer. *New Eng. J. Med.* 294:405, 1976.

Culliton, B.J. Breast cancer: Reports of new therapy are greatly exaggerated. *Science* 191:1029, 1976.

Cutler, S.J., Christine, B., Barclay, T.H.C. Increasing incidence and decreasing mortality rates for breast cancer. *Cancer* 28:1376, 1971.

Egan, R.L. Evolution of the team approach in breast cancer. *Cancer* 36:1815, 1975.

Egan, R.L. Bilateral breast carcinomas. Role of mammography. *Cancer* 38:931, 1976.

Egan, R.L., Ellis, J.T., Powell, R.W. Team approach to the study of diseases of the breast. *Cancer* 23:847, 1969.

Fisher, B. Cooperative clinical trials in primary breast cancer: A critical appraisal. *Cancer* 31, 1271, 1973.

Fisher, B., Carbone, P., Economou, S.G., Frelick, R., Glass, A., Lerner, H., Redmond, C., Zelen, M., Band, P., Katrych, D.L., Wolmark, N., Fisher, E.R. 1-Phenylalanine mustard (L-PAM) in the management of primary breast cancer. A report of early findings. *New Eng. J. Med.* 292:117, 1975.

Fisher, E.R. Ultrastructure of the human breast and its disorders. *Am. J. Clin. Path.* 66:291, 1976.

Fisher, E.R., Posada, H., Ramos, H. Evaluation of mammography based upon correlation of specimen mammograms and histopathologic findings. *Am. J. Clin. Path.* 62:60, 1974.

Fukami, A., Kasumi, F., Hori, M., Kuno, K., Kajitani, T., Sakamoto, G., Sugano, H. Bilateral primary breast cancer treated at the Cancer Institute Hospital, Tokyo, In *Breast Cancer.* Montague, A.C.W. Stonesifer, G.L., Jr., Lewison, E.F. (eds.) New York: Alan R. Liss, 1977, pp. 525-535.

Gallager, H.S. Breast specimen radiography. Obligatory, adjuvant and investigative. *Am. J. Clin. Path.* 64:749, 1975.

Gallager, H.S. Treatment selection in primary breast cancer. Pathologic considerations. *Am. J. Roentgenol.* 126:135, 1976.

Gallager, H.S., Martin, J.E. The study of mammary carcinoma by mammography and whole organ sectioning. Early observations. *Cancer* 23:855, 1969.

Gallager, H.S., Martin, J.E. An orientation to the concept of minimal breast cancer. *Cancer* 28:1505, 1971.

Goldenberg, V.E., Goldenberg, N.S., Sommers, S.C. Comparative ultrastructure of atypical ductal hyperplasia, intraductal carcinoma, and infiltrating ductal carcinoma of the breast. *Cancer* 24:1152, 1969.

Greenwald, P., Nasca, P.C., Lawrence, C.E., Horton, J., McGarrah, R.P., Gabriele, T., Carlton, K. Estimated effect of breast self-examination and routine physician examinations on breast-cancer mortality. *New Eng. J. Med.* 299:271, 1978.

Gullino, P.M. Considerations on the preneoplastic lesions of the mammary gland. *Am. J. Pathol.* 89:413, 1977.

Hajdu, S.I., Melamed, M.E. The diagnostic value of aspiration smears. *Am. J. Clin. Path.* 59:350, 1973.

Horowitz, K.B., McGuire, W.L. Estrogen and progesterone: Their relationship in hormone-dependent breast cancer, In *Progesterone Receptors in Normal and Neoplastic Tissues.* McGuire, W.L., Raynaud, J.P., Baulieu, E.E. (eds.). New York: Raven Press, 1977, pp. 103-124.

Hutter, R.V.P. The pathologist's role in minimal breast cancer. *Cancer* 28:1527, 1971.

Jensen, H.M., Wellings, S.R. Preneoplastic lesions of the human mammary gland transplanted into the nude athymic mouse. *Cancer Res.* 36:2605, 1976.

Koehl, R.H., Snyder, R.E., Hutter, R.V.P., Foote, F.W. The incidence and significance of calcifications within operative breast specimens. *Am. J. Clin. Path.* 53:3, 1970.

Lagios, M.D. Multicentricity of breast carcinoma demonstrated by routine correlated serial subgross and radiographic examination. *Cancer* 40:1726, 1977.

Leis, H.P., Jr., Mersheimer, W.L., Black, M.M., and Chabon, A.B. The second breast. *New York State J. Med.* 65:2460, 1965.

Lippman, M.E., Allegra, J.C., Thompson, E.B., Simon, R., Barlock, A., Green, L., Huff, K.K., Do, H.M.T., Aitken, S.C., Warren, R. The relation between estrogen receptors and response rate to cytotoxic chemotherapy in metastatic breast cancer. *New Eng. J. Med.* 298:1223, 1978.

Ludwig, A.S., Okagaki, T., Richart, R.M., Lattes, R. Nuclear DNA content of lobular carcinoma *in situ* of the breast. *Cancer* 31:1553, 1973.

McDivitt, R.W. Progress in human pathology. Breast carcinoma. *Human Pathology* 9:3, 1978.

McGuire, W.L., Carbone, P.P., Sears, M.E., Escher, G.C. Estrogen receptors in human breast cancer: An overview. In *Estrogen Receptors in Human Breast Cancer,* McGuire, W.L., Carbone, P.P., Vollmer, E.P. (eds.), New York: Raven Press, 1975, pp. 1-7.

McGuire, W.L., Horowitz, K.B., Pearson, O.H., Segaloff, A. Current status of estrogen and progesterone receptors in breast cancer. *Cancer* 39:2934, 1977.

Murad, T.M. Ultrastructure of ductular carcinoma of the breast (*in situ* and infiltrating lobular carcinoma). *Cancer* 27:18, 1971.

Ozello, L. Ultrastructure of intra-epithelial carcinomas of the breast. *Cancer* 28,1508, 1971.

Ozello, L., Sanpitak, P. Epithelial-stromal junction of intraductal carcinoma of the breast. *Cancer* 26, 1186, 1970.

Pertschuk, L.P., Tobin, E.H., Brigati, D.J., Kim, D.S., Bloom, N.D., Gaetjens, E., Berman, P.J., Carter, A.C., Degenshein, G.A. Immunofluorescent detection of estrogen receptors in breast cancer. Comparison with dextran-coated charcoal and sucrose gradient assays. *Cancer* 41:907, 1978.

Rosen, P.P., Lieberman, P.H., Braun, D.W., Jr., Kosloff, C., Adair, F. Lobular carcinoma *in situ* of the breast. Detailed analysis of 99 patients with average follow-up of 24 years. *Am. J. Surg. Path.* 2:225, 1978.

Rosen, P.P., Snyder, R.E., Foote, F.W., Wallace, R.T. Detection of occult carcinoma in the apparently benign breast biopsy through specimen radiography. *Cancer* 26, 944, 1970.

Rosen, P.P., Snyder, R.E., Robbins, G. Specimen radiography for non palpable breast lesions found by mammography: Procedures and results. *Cancer* 34:2028, 1974.

Scarff, R.W., Torloni, H. Histologic typing of breast tumors, In *International Histologic Classification of Tumors* (No. 2). Geneva: World Health Organization, 1968, pp. 1-20.

Schottenfeld, D., Nash, A.G., Robbins, G.F., Beattie, E.J. Ten-year results of treatment of primary operable breast carcinoma. A summary of 304 patients evaluated by the TNM system. *Cancer* 38:1001, 1976.

Schwartz, G.F., Feig, S.A., Patchefsky, A.S. Clinico-pathologic correlations and significance of clinically occult mammary lesions. *Cancer* 41:1147, 1978.

Snyder, R.E., Rosen, P.P. Radiography of breast specimens. *Cancer* 28:1608, 1971.

Terenius, L., Johansson, H., Rimsten, A., Thorén, L. Malignant and benign human mammary disease: Estrogen binding in relation to clinical data. *Cancer* 33:1364, 1974.

Urban, J.A. Changing patterns of breast cancer. Lucy Wortham James Lecture (Clinical). *Cancer* 37:111, 1976.

Urban, J.A. Changing patterns of breast cancer. *Bull. N.Y. Acad. Med.* 53:749, 1977.

Urban, J.A. Bilateral breast cancer.—Biopsy of contralateral breast. In *Breast Cancer.* Montague, A.C.W., Stonesifer, G.L., Jr., Lewison, E.F., (eds.). New York: Alan R. Liss, 1977A, pp. 517-523.

Urban, J.A., Papachristou, D., Taylor, J. Bilateral breast cancer. Biopsy of the opposite breast. *Cancer* 40:1968, 1977.

Wellings, S.R., Jensen, H.M., Marcum, R.G. An atlas of subgross pathology of the human breast with special reference to possible precancerous lesions. *J. Natl. Cancer Inst.* 55:231, 1975.

Wolfe, J.N. Risk for breast cancer development determined by mammographic parenchymal pattern. *Cancer* 37:2486, 1976.

Zajdela, A., Ghossein, N.A., Pilleron, J.P., Ennuyer, A. The value of aspiration cytology in the diagnosis of breast cancer: Experience at the Foundation Curie. *Cancer* 35:499, 1975.

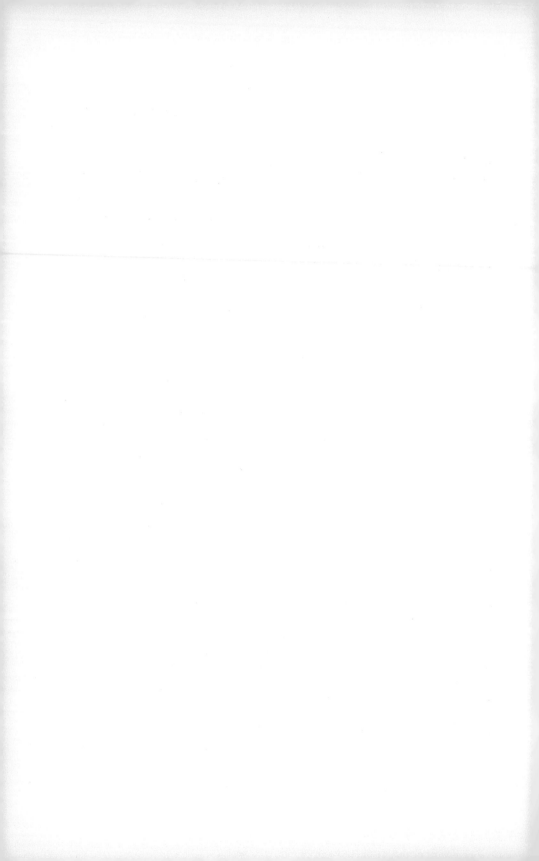

CHAPTER 8

The Surgery of Breast Cancer

PETER I. PRESSMAN

THE SURGEON'S ROLE

The primary treatment of breast cancer is surgical. The diagnosis may be suspected either on the basis of a finding on physical examination or the presence of an abnormality on x-ray, but tissue must be obtained and examined under the microscope by a pathologist before treatment is instituted. The surgical biopsy is the means by which a diagnosis is established and is the first phase of any plan of treatment. Since cancer of the breast is rare in men, for whom treatment of the primary tumor is similar to that in women, it is cancer of the female breast which is discussed.

Surgery is the modality most commonly used to treat breast cancer and there are four goals for which a definitive surgical procedure is performed:

1) To cure the patient so that she will survive without the development of disseminated disease.

2) To accomplish control of the disease on the chest wall and in the axilla so as to prevent local and regional recurrence in both patients who are cured and in those who develop disseminated disease.

3) To stage the disease by obtaining adequate tissues in order to determine whether adjunctive chemotherapy or radiation is indicated, and to establish the hormonal status of the tumor.

4) To leave the patient cosmetically, physically, and psychologically as near normal as possible.

Of these four goals, to cure the patient is obviously the most important, but all of these goals should be integrated in planning treatment.

The surgeon plays a pivotal role in the diagnosis and treatment of a patient with breast cancer. This role commences with deciding to do a biopsy and planning the pre- and postoperative workup, and, of course, continues in performing the surgery which has been recommended to and accepted by the patient.

The approach becomes multidisciplinary when the pathology report is complete, and the results are interpreted by the surgeon. It is usually at this phase that the oncologist and radiotherapist become a part of the team in order to plan further treatment. However, in certain instances, such as when the patient in clinical Stage III or IV of breast cancer has had an obvious diagnosis, the consultants should work together preoperatively. If no adjunctive therapies are recommended it should be the responsibility of the surgeon to follow the patient for the remainder of her life. Even if radiation, chemotherapy, or hormonal modalities are employed, it is the surgeon who should remain responsible for orchestrating the necessary treatment. This should include an awareness which patients may benefit from psychiatric help and which patients may be candidates for reconstructive surgery if it seems appropriate.

DETECTION BY MAMMOGRAPHY

The majority of breast cancers are detected by physical examination of the breasts, either on self-examination by the patient or by her physician. Where x-rays of the breasts are performed as a part of a program of screening asymptomatic women, mammography has added significantly to the detection of breast cancer at a stage before palpation of a mass is possible. When it is employed diagnostically it must be remembered that its accuracy does not substitute for a biopsy of a palpable lesion. Because of the highly publicized results of screening mammography, many physicians and their patients have come to rely on a negative x-ray report as assurance that no malignancy is present. With an increaaasing dependence on the x-ray study, there has been reluctance to perform biopsies without an x-ray confirmation of a malignancy. Subtle lesions that have been detected have enlarged before surgical biopsy was recommended because of the false sense of security afforded by an x-ray examination, which yielded a report on a lesion as either negative or benign.

A study of 100 consecutive patients who were operated on for breast cancer and who were examined preoperatively either by mammography or xeroradiography has been reported (Pressman, 1977). Actually, 106 cancers were included in this study, because six patients were proven to have simultaneous bilateral breast malignancies. The x-ray examinations were done by radiologists in different settings—hospitals, screening centers for breast cancer, offices of general radiology practitioners and offices of physicians specializing in mammography.

The study showed that 59% of the cancers were correctly identified by x-ray, 31% were negative studies and 10% were described as benign lesions. There were 12 patients whose treatment was delayed from three to 12 months because mammography had not identified the malignancy, although, a clinical abnormality had been present. Only when the palpable tumors were observed to enlarge clinically were the patients referred for biopsy. At the time the biopsies were performed, three of these patients were inoperable, five patients were found to have extensive axillary metastases and three patients had one to two lymph nodes involved. Only two patients did not have lymph node involvement and subsequently both have developed metastatic disease and have died. It is of particular interest that these were both women in their twenties who were considered by their physicians to have fibroadenomas that did not require excision. In all of these cases the patients and their physicians had been reassured on the basis of the mammography that no serious pathology existed, although a clinical abnormality had been present.

The 59% accuracy rate of diagnostic mammography in this study may not be the best that can be achieved, but since the x-ray studies were performed in varied settings, these results are considered to reflect those of common practice in this community. When a lump has been found in the breast, a negative finding or the description of a benign lesion based on diagnostic mammography, must not provide a false sense of security to the physician. Diagnostic mammography is an adjunctive method to physical examination; it does not rule out the presence of a cancer and must not substitute for biopsy of a palpable lesion.

BIOPSY

By definition, a biopsy is "the gross and microscopic examination of tissues removed from the body as an aid to medical diagnosis" (Morris, 1969). Whether the biopsy should be excisional or incisional should depend on the suspected findings and the size of the lesion. A large malignant tumor is more easily incised, whereas, benign tumors and smaller lesions can be completely removed.

It is often less traumatic and neater to completely remove a large segment of breast tissue to include the suspected malignancy rather than to seek out the tumor mass, incise it, and have to suture the rigid walls of a carcinoma to control bleeding. Whatever the setting in which the biopsy is performed, it is important to provide an adequate amount of tissue, not only to establish the diagnosis of malignancy, but to obtain estrogen and progesterone receptor assays on the specimen. Because of the proven value of the assays in predicting hormonal responsiveness if metastases should occur at a future date, obtaining the assays should be as routine as obtaining a pathologic diagnosis prior to a mastectomy. The tissues must be immediately frozen, because the receptor protein is extremely heat labile.

There has been increasing interest in separating the initial biopsy from the mastectomy itself—performing it as a separate operative procedure at a different time. Psychiatrists and some women patients have urged that this be done. According to the available studies, it is not harmful—that is, there is no demonstrable adverse effect on the eventual cure by delaying definitive surgery up to two weeks (Abramson, 1976). But the biopsy must be undertaken with the understanding that definitive treatment, either surgery or radiation, will then be initiated.

Performing a preliminary biopsy does have the advantage of identifying those women who have a malignancy so that bone scanning can be done, and unnecessary comprehensive workups can be avoided on the larger number of patients who ultimately will prove to have benign disease. Psychologically, this is an enormous advantage particularly for those women who will not require further surgery.

The ultimate gain is realized when the biopsy can be done on an outpatient basis. This saves hospital beds, eases operating schedules, and is less costly to the patient. Outpatient surgery usually means administering local anesthesia. The limitations of local anesthesia must be recognized, however; its use makes it more difficult for the surgeon to do his work—to be meticulous and to maintain patient comfort. Poorly defined lesions cannot be explored, and deeply placed tumors might well be missed. Small, superficial, and well circumscribed tumors are amenable to the technique of local anesthesia. When lesions are firm and superficial, even if there is a suspicion of a malignancy, they can be safely removed with the patient under local anesthesia. One tremendous advantage to this technique is that tiny lesions that might otherwise be observed until they enlarge can be removed sooner because of the ease of this procedure and its acceptance by patients. patients.

More extensive surgical procedures are required to excise poorly defined masses and to seek out non-palpable lesions detected by mammography, such as microcalcifications. General anesthesia is necessary, and these operations can be performed with patients on an ambulatory basis, only in special units where this can be provided.

Finally, it is important to state that there are many patients and surgeons who prefer to have the biopsy performed under a general anesthetic with a frozen section and an immediate mastectomy. all of which has been discussed preoperatively. This is preferred by some women who do not want to have a separate biopsy that will necessitate a second operation. We offer the option for these approaches to the patient. In two situations we encourage separate procedures—when small superficial lesions can be excised under local anesthesia, and when microcalcifications are sought by the pathologist, who will probably require multiple specimens and permanent sections to establish a definitive diagnosis.

SURGICAL PROCEDURES

Since the early part of this century the most commonly performed surgical procedure for operable breast cancer has been the standard radical mastectomy. Only in the past two decades have other surgical procedures been gaining acceptance, and the indications for their use in the treatment of potentially curable breast cancer becoming clearer. The operations I will describe are listed in Table I.

Table I.
Surgical Procedures

1. Standard radical mastectomy.
2. Extended radical mastectomy (Urban).
3. Modified radical mastectomy (Patey).
4. Extended simple mastectomy (Auchincloss).
5. Total (simple) mastectomy.
6. Partial mastectomy.
7. Subcutaneous mastectomy.

The standard radical mastectomy, described by Halsted in 1894 and popularized in this century by Dr. Cushman Haagensen, is designed to remove the skin of the protuberant breast with skin flaps which are developed to the clavicle, to the midline of the sternum, to the lowest ribs, and toward the latissimus dorsi laterally. The procedure consists of an en bloc removal of the breast, the pectoralis major and minor muscles, and a dissection of the axillary contents.

Because of the wide area of skin removed in the classic operation, skin grafting is frequently required. The cure rate and minimal local recurrence achieved by this procedure have become standards by which other methods of treatment are measured (Haagensen, 1971). It is a deforming operation because removal of the pectoralis major muscle creates a deep cleft between the arm and the chest wall. Many surgeons performing this operation today preserve enough skin so that skin grafting is not required.

There are several techniques for anatomically extending the radical mastectomy. The best known is the Urban procedure, in which an en bloc resection of the internal mammary chain of lymph nodes augments the standard radical mastectomy (Urban, 1959). This extended technique can be employed when a cancer is located in the parasternal or subareolar region, because of the frequency of involvement of the internal mammary nodes.

The operation that has become more frequently used and which, in many institutions, has supplanted the radical mastectomy entirely is the modified radical mastectomy. Modified radical mastectomy is a term that describes a spectrum of operative procedures since the extent of dissection varies considerably. The extent of tissue removal depends on the surgeon's philosophy involved in selecting the operation as well as on his surgical expertise. Sometimes the surgery is badly performed, being little more than removal of a few nodes that can be pulled down from beneath the pectoralis muscles and divided at the end of a total mastectomy. If, however, it is the intent of the surgeon to do a complete axillary dissection, the pectoralis minor muscle can be removed and the inter-pectoral tissues dissected so as to remain with the specimen. Aided by upward rotation of the patient's arm, a meticulous and nearly complete axillary dissection in continuity can be accomplished. When this is done the procedure is known as the Patey modification of the radical mastectomy. It also has been called the conservative radical mastectomy, because it is basically a radical mastectomy with preservation of the pectoralis major muscle. This accomplishes the aim of a radical mastectomy without the deformity.

In another approach to performing a modified radical mastectomy, both pectoral muscles are preserved. This is a total mastectomy with lower axillary dissection, as described by Auchincloss, 1963). Another term for this procedure is an extended simple mastectomy. While the lowest levels of the axillary lymph nodes can always be removed, it may not be nearly as complete an axillary dissection as any of the previously described procedures can be.

Over the past several decades, substituting a modified radical mastectomy for the standard radical mastectomy has been considered the conservative approach. Recently, the term conservatism has come to mean even less extensive surgery than that of a modified radical mastectomy. These two operations are the total mastectomy and the partial mastectomy.

Total mastectomy is the operation, which until recently has been called the simple mastectomy. The term should really be total or complete mastectomy, because in this operation the skin flaps are developed in exactly the same manner as is done in the radical mastectomy. The pectoralis major fascia is also removed along with the axillary tail of the breast. If the removal of the breast is total, an average of three to seven axillary lymph nodes will frequently be found by the pathologist when the specimen is carefully examined. I advise a total mastectomy when a diagnosed carcinoma is noninvasive. In this situation the chance of lymph node involvement is under 1%. In the course of the operation the axilla can be explored and any enlarged or firm lymph nodes can be removed and examined by the pathologist with a frozen section. If unsuspected metastases are encountered, a total axillary dissection can be performed, converting the operation into a modified radical mastectomy.

Partial mastectomy, also known as segmental resection or segmental mastectomy, means removal of a part of the breast, usually a full thickness quadrant, which includes the skin and underlying msucle fascia with primary closure of the defect. This is not a "lumpectomy," which means simple enucleation of the tumor and plays no role in cancer surgery other than that of an excisional biopsy, which it actually is. The partial mastectomy does leave the patient with a smaller breast. Depending on the size of the patient's breast and the location of the tumor, the remaining breast may be grossly deformed by this procedure.

The subcutaneous mastectomy is not considered to be a true cancer operation. In this procedure an incision is usually made beneath the breast and proceeding upward from below, the breast tissue is excised. Comparing this with the total mastectomy described above, it is obvious that not only is the nipple undisturbed by the subcutaneous mastectomy, but it is almost impossible to totally remove the axillary prolongation of the breast and the ductal structures beneath the nipple so that the nipple will survive. Breast tissue does remain after a subcutaneous mastectomy, and breast cancer has developed in these remnants. Thus, this procedure does not achieve what the total mastectomy can accomplish.

What is the role for a more conservative approach to breast surgery? It is the result of changing concepts of the disease and also of detection of breast cancer at an earlier time in its natural history. In 1863 when James Paget wrote that he was not aware of a single instance of a patient living for 10 years following surgical treatmet of breast cancer, he was describing simple excision of breast tumors that were usually large.

The next generation of surgeons attacked the disease more aggressively and developed more extensive operations. Long-term survival was sometimes achieved, but there was a local recurrence rate of 65%. In 1882, Halsted began performing the radical mastectomy and he emphasized the need to sacrifice a much greater area of skin over the breast which always necessitated skin grafting. By 1894 he was able to report that of 50 patients who had radical mastectomies, only three had local recurrences.

It is interesting to note that Halsted designed his operation based on the prevailing concept of the biology of breast cancer of his time. There was little significance placed on the blood stream as a mechanism for developing metastases. The pathologists of that era believed that cancer of the breast spread in a centrifugal manner, usually in continuity with the original growth, permeating all organs by the lymphatics and along fascial planes, rather than disseminating via the blood stream. It was felt that tumor emboli in venous channels were thrombosed and trapped and did not metastasize. It is as a result of this concept of tumor behavior that Halsted formulated the surgical principles that have had an enduring impact on surgery for breast cancer. It is remarkable that although the radical mastectomy was based on an incomplete understanding of the behavior of the disease, it has proven to be an excellent operation for the treatment of early breast cancer.

While the radical mastectomy was the single most important contribution of the early part of this century, mammography has contributed to changing the surgical approach more recently. With the ability to detect cancers before they become palpable and frequently without involvement of the axillary lymph nodes, clinicians can treat malignancies at an earlier time in their natural history, and patients may be cured with a less extensive operation. Each of the operative procedures described above has a place in certain patients, according to the type and stage of the disease. I recommend the Patey type of modified radical mastectomy and perform it most frequently as the operation of choice for operable, infiltrating breast cancer. I also perform a contralateral breast biopsy at the time of the mastectomy.

There has been an increasing awareness of the multicentricity of breast cancer, and this is the rationale for total breast removal if an invasive cancer is diagnosed. We have learned from our pathologists that when detailed studies of mastectomy specimens are performed, the reported incidence of multicentric malignancy is 25% to 45% (Gallager and Martin, 1969). In all probability, failure of partial mastectomy and lumpectomy to control breast cancer locally is related to this multicentric occurrence of breast cancer. Thus, this is the rationale for total breast removal if an invasive cancer is diagnosed.

Multicentricity has also been a stimulus for interest in the contralateral breast. A woman who has had a mastectomy is at the highest risk for developing cancer in the remaining breast. One can expect that 15% of patients who survive 10 years following a mastectomy for breast cancer in the course of the clinical follow-up will develop a new cancer (Urban, 1959). Unfortunately, the second primary breast cancer is frequently seen in a more advanced stage than the one for which the patient had been treated successfully and determines the fate of the patient. With a biopsy of the contralateral breast at the time of the mastectomy, it is possible to detect occult breast cancer in an earlier stage of development. Urban reported that 12.5% of these breast biopsies contain carcinoma. To evaluate the reproductability of this finding, I performed 85 consecutive contralateral biopsies at the time of mastectomy. Twelve patients were found to have bilateral breast cancer (14%)—two on minimal clinical suspicion and 10 (12%) on random biopsy—in the absence of clinical or radiographic findings (Pressman, 1979).

When performing the random biopsy, any palpable thickening of the contralateral breast or questionable finding on mammography deserves investigation. The use of a mirror image and/or the upper outer quadrant of the breast statistically have provided the most productive location to perform a generous contralateral biopsy. I use circumareolar incisions to enter the breast tissue. By preserving the subcutaneous fat of the breast, one can obtain a large amount of breast tissue extending out toward the quadrant of the palpable tumor. If the mirror image is the upper outer quadrant of the breast, a paramammary or oblique incision can be employed and again, by preserving the subcutaneous tissues of the breast, a generous segment of breast parenchyma can be removed without producing breast deformity or unsightly scars.

It is in patients in whom an occult, noninvasive carcinoma is found that a total mastectomy with lower axillary dissection is an adequate operation. When cancer of the breast is invasive, an axillary dissection should be performed. If we could know with certainty that a particular patient with breast cancer had no axillary lymph node involvement, there would be no reason to perform a lymph node dissection. It is well known that there is an error rate of approximately 35% in clinically judging whether axillary lymph nodes are involved. Even at the time of operation, direct palpation of the axillary nodes and random biopsy are not enough for an accurate diagnosis. We know from our daily experience that we are frequently surprised to find that what appear to be normal nodes contain carcinoma when we examined them microscopically. If a total mastectomy alone is done in such cases, microscopic cancer can be left behind.

It has been reported that when patients have micrometastases alone, particularly if only Level I is involved their prognosis is similar to that of patients with pathologic Stage I cancer (Atteyeh, 1977). Thus, removal of the axillary lymph nodes has a therapeutic value because nodes containing cancer are excised. The question of interfering with immunologic competence by removing lymph nodes, I feel, can be answered as follows: If a tumor has metastasized to the axillary lymph nodes, the competence of these nodes is proven inadequate. As far as any systemic immune response, all of which is theoretical, this should be shared by the remaining lymph nodal areas.

In summary, at this time probably the most commonly performed operation and the best conceived, based on our current knowledge, is a surgical procedure that includes total breast removal and an axillary dissection. This removes the entire tumor-bearing breast and the lymph nodes that may harbor metastases. Biopsies of the internal mammary lymph nodes when the cancers are medially located, can provide additional information for planning therapy. The contralateral biopsy is an additional means of earlier detection of breast cancer in a high risk population (patients with cancer of the breast).

An awareness of the presence and location of lymph node metastases makes it possible to stage the disease not only to determine the prognosis but also to plan adjunctive therapy. Most patients with negative axillary lymph nodes will be cured of their disease by surgical means alone. We know that there is a linear relationship between local recurrence and the magnitude of lymph node involvement. Radiation therapy and chemotherapy reduce local recurrence. In certain situations, such as medially located carcinomas, the axillary lymph nodes alone may not provide enough information. If they are proven by frozen section to be positive in the course of an axillary dissection, there is a high probability of internal mammary nodal involvement. If the axillary nodes are considered benign, however, by performing biopsies of the internal mammary nodes important information is obtained. If the biopsy is positive, there is an indication for adjuvant chemotherapy and/or radiation therapy to the internal mammary chain, assuming gross disease remains. Some surgeons prefer to treat this nodal chain with radiation routinely in medial lesions. I recommend that that biopsies of the nodes be taken in order to aid in selecting patients for adjuvant chemotherapy.

Two lesser operations have been widely publicized in the media and are frequently requested by patients. The first of these is the lumpectomy, which is a wide excisional biopsy. This method was recommended several years ago by Dr. George Crile, of the Cleveland Clinic, for apparently localized breast cancer in women who refused mastectomy. These patients have now been followed for over five years, and the results have been unacceptable, as judged by the recurrence rate and poor suvival in patients classified as having Stage I and II cancers. This approach has been abandoned at the Cleveland Clinic, where the modified radical mastectomy is recommended instead.

The other minimal surgical procedure is the partial mastectomy. This has been advocated as part of an approach that includes radiation therapy and, at times, chemotherapy (Cope, 1976). Following a biopsy to determine the diagnosis, a partial mastectomy is performed followed by an axillary dissection, in continuity if feasible and discontinuous if necessary. The purpose of this operation is to perform a wide excision of the breast cancer and to stage the disease with regard to the axillary lymph nodes. Radiation therapy is then employed to treat the remaining breast and adjuvant chemotherapy is administered if there is demonstrated lymph node involvement or microscopic blood vessel invasion.

While this is an intriguing multidisciplinary approach there are many problems. Partial mastectomy can produce an extremely deformed breast. Some patients have required subsequent mastectomies, and the complications related to radiation therapy have been high. Additionally, particularly if this approach is used in young women, one does not know what the long-term effects will be on the remaining breast tissue, which has been irradiated, in those patients who are cured of disease.

Finally, one must always individualize treatment. For the patient who will not agree to a mastectomy, there are other promising approaches that are being tested in clinical trials throughout the world and that can be applied with good conscience in individual cases.

ABLATIVE SURGERY

In all probability hormones are not an initiating factor in the formation of a breast cancer. The role of hormones in stimulating the growth of cancer of the breast, however, has been known for 80 years. Beatsen (1896) demonstrated that oophorectomy could induce remission of advanced breast cancer in premenopausal females. Adrenalectomy was introduced in 1951 (Huggins et al.) to control metastatic breast carcinoma in postmenopausal women, and the success of the procedure provided additional evidence that certain breast carcinomas are hormonally dependent. Hypophysectomy produces results similar to those of bilateral adrenalectomy and completes our understanding of the existence of a pituitary-adrenal-ovarian axis. Adrenalectomy is the more commonly peformed procedure, because it has been safe in the hands of many surgeons and because replacement therapy requires only cortisone.

It has been apparent that breast carcinomas are either hormone-dependent or independent. Those that are not hormone-dependent are called autonomous, they are unaffected by hormonal therapy and by ablative procedures. Those carcinomas that are hormonally responsive *are* affected by either additive hormonal therapies, such as the administration of male or female hormones or anti-estrogens, and by ablative procedures such as adrenalectomy or oophorectomy.

Selecting patients whose tumors are likely to respond is, obviously, important. Applying a constellation of clinical criteria, approximately 35% of premenopausal patients with recurrent breast cancer can be expected to respond to oophorectomy, and a similar percentage of postmenopausal patients to adrenalectomy. A combined adrenalectomy-oophorectomy is often performed in premenopausal (and recently postmenopausal) patients to maximize the potential for response.

It is important to emphasize that interest in ablative procedures has remained high for 80 years because the palliation accomplished in individual patients is frequently dramatic and is often sustained for many months or years. More important the quality of life for these patients is excellent. Replacement therapy consists of administering oral cortisone acetate (37.5 mg to 50 mg a day); at this minute dosage there are none of the side effects of steroid therapy. Responders survive longer than non-responders. An objective response has always been defined as a decrease by 50% in the size of measurable lesions, which is sustained for at least six months.

One of the most significant developments in the treatment of breast cancer has been the in vitro assay for hormonal receptors (Jensen, 1971). Cytoplasmic protein in membrane receptor sites have been identified, and it is apparent that those patients who respond have tumors that contain estrogen receptor protein. Tumors lacking in or are weak in estrogen receptor (ER) continue to grow autonomously and are not considered responsive tumors. Approximately one third of breast cancers are hormone-dependent, as had been suspected on the basis of previous empirical clinical experience.

In 1974 the Breast Cancer Task Force of the National Cancer Institute reported the clinical correlation between ER binding and the response to ablative procedures (Jensen, 1971). In a group of 274 patients who had surgical ablation, the overall rate of objective tumor regression was 32%. A response rate of 58% was achieved in those patients whose tumors had positive ER values, whereas only a 5% response rate was found in patients whose tumors were ER negative.

This ability to predict the response rate to a therapeutic modality, based on an in vitro laboratory assay, represents a tremendous advance. Predictability is not possible with chemotherapeutic agents at this time.

It is intriguing that some ER-positive tumors fail to respond. Some information has been acquired to explain this. On the whole, the receptor status of the primary breast cancer, assayed at the time of mastectomy, is retained. Hormonal dependence, however, may be lost as the disease progresses; 10% fewer metastases are estrogen receptor-positive than is the primary tumor. The estrogen receptor assay is also not an all-or-none phenomenon; it is a quantitative test using measures of fentomoles per milligram of protein. A tumor with 10 fentomoles has estrogen receptor protein, as does a tumor with 1,000. The response differs according to the number of fentomoles.

In human tissue culture, the estrogen receptor regulates the progesterone receptor (PGR), and there is a direct linear relationship between high estrogen and progesterone receptors. Only rarely is the progesterone receptor present in the absence of estrogen receptor, and this is not well understood. Where both ER and PGR are present, a response rate of 86% following surgical ablation has been reported (Degenshein, et al., 1977). The best response rates can be expected if patient selection for ablation includes consideration of clinical criteria in addition to the laboratory assay. These criteria are a long disease-free interval and predominantly osseous or pleural metastases.

Obtaining hormonal receptors should be as routine as preparing the frozen section when a biopsy of the breast is performed. While a needle biopsy can be performed to support the suspicion of malignancy, I recommend that in all stages of breast malignancy an adequate surgical biopsy be performed to establish the diagnosis histologically, not only to obviate cytological errors, but in order to obtain tissue for receptor testing. The information thus gained is vital in planning therapy for those patients who ultimately prove to have recurrent disease.

While ablative surgery has been used mainly in metastatic disease, it has been demonstrated that it can be an important primary modality of treatment in inflammatory cancer (Yonemoto, et al., 1970). There are recent reports that indicate that it is a useful approach as part of a combined therapeutic regimen in Stage III breast cancer, probably because most patients in this category are really undiagnosed Stage IV patients when they are treated (Bland, et al., 1975). The recent data from adjunctive chemotherapy studies suggest that there may be an important hormonal effect of the cytotoxic drugs in premenopausal women. In the future, the use of hormonal assays, along with endocrine ablation may be recommended for post-mastectomy patients who are at high risk for developing recurrent disease and whose tumors are ER and PGR positive (Dao et al., 1975).

We have used as our indication for performing an adrenalectomy the development of advancing metastatic disease in patients whose hormonal receptors have been measured as positive either by tumor assay at the time of the initial mastectomy or biopsy of a metastatic site. Adrenalectomy is performed on those patients who have had an objective response to oophorectomy. A combined adrenalectomy-oophrectomy is preferred for premenopausal patients who are near menopause, for all postmenopausal patients, and for younger women in whom the progression of metastases is considered virulent.

It is mandatory that the procedure be made as safe as possible and also that surgical exploration provide information about the extent of intra-abdominal metastatic disease so that adjunctive therapy can be planned. Adrenalectomy has been traditionally performed either anteriorly, via an abdominal incision, or posteriorly, via bilateral flank incisions. Each approach has its own characteristic complications, which are responsible for morbidity. Since this is an elective surgical procedure directed toward palliation, acceptable mortality and morbidity rates should be close to zero.

I have reported the experience at the Beth Israel Hospital Medical Center and described a transabdominal technique, which has achieved these goals. I recommend the abdominal approach not only because it has been entirely safe, but because the oophorectomy can be performed via the same upper abdominal transverse incision, and a thorough exploration and staging of the extent of the disease can be achieved (Pressman, 1976).

It is anticipated that more adrenalectomies will be performed earlier in the course of metastatic disease, because it can be recommended to suitable candidates with confidence. In those patients who can be expected to respond, this modality can be the first approach to treating recurrent and metastatic breast cancer. Chemotherapy and radiation can be added when the remission has ceased.

REFERENCES

Abramson, D.J. Delayed mastectomy after outpatient biopsy. *Amer. J. Surg.* 132:596, 1976.

Attiyeh, F.A., Jensen, M., Huvos, A.G., Fracchia, A. Axillary micrometastasis and macrometastasis in carcinoma of the breast. *Surg. Gynec., and Obst.* 144:839, 1977.

Auchincloss, H. Significance of location and number of axillary metastases in carcinoma of the breast: A justification for a conservative operation. *Ann. Surg.* 158:37, 1963.

Beatson, G.T. On the treatment of inoperable cases of carcinoma: suggestions for a new method of treatment with illustrative cases. *Lancet* 2:104, 1896.

Bland, K.I., O'Leary, J.P., Woodward, E.R., Dragstedt, L.R. Immediate oophorectomy and adrenalectomy in the treatment of Stage III breast carcinoma. *Amer. J. Surg.* 129:277, 1975.

Cope, O., Wang, C.A., Chu, A., eta al. Limited surgical excision as the basis of a comprehensive therapy for cancer of the breast. *Amer. J. Surg.* 131:400, 1976.

Dao, T.L., Nemoto, T., Chamberlain, A. Bross, I. Adrenalectomy with radical mastectomy in the treatment of high risk breast cancer. *Cancer* 35:487, 1975.

Degenshein, G.A., Bloom, N., Ceccarelli, F., Daluvoy, R., Tobin, E. Estrogen and progesterone receptor site studies as guides to the management of advanced breast cancer. *Breast* 3:, 1977.

Gallager, H.S., Martin, J. Early phases in the development of breast cancer. *Cancer* 24:1170, 1969.

Haagensen, C., Diseases of the breast. Philadelphia: W.B. Saunders Company, 1971.

Huggins, C., Bergenstal, D.M. Inhibition of human mammary and prostatic cancer by adrenalectomy. *Cancer Res.* 12:134, 1952.

Jensen, E.V., Block, G.E., Smith, S., et al. Estrogen receptors and breast cancer response to adrenalectomy in prediction of response in cancer therapy. National Cancer Institute Monograph No. 34 Hall, T.C. (ed.) pp. 55-70. Washington, D.C.: U.S. Government Printing Office, 1971.

Morris, W. *The American Heritage Dictionary of the English Language.* p. 133. Boston: American Heritage Publishing, 1969.

Pressman, P.I. Technique of adrenalectomy for metastatic breast cancer. *Surg. Gynec., and Obst.* 142:743, 1976.

Pressman, P.I. Mammography in surgical practice. *Amer. J. Surg.* 133:702, 1977.

Pressman, P.I. Bilateral breast cancer: the contralateral breast biopsy. *Breast v. 5* 3:29-33, 1979.

Urban, J.A. Clinical experience and results of excision of the internal mammary lymph node chain in primary operable breast cancer. *Cancer* 12:14, 1959.

Yonemoto, R.H., Keating, J.L., Byron, R.L., Riihimaki, D.U. Inflammatory carcinoma of the breast treated by bilateral adrenalectomy. *Surgery* 68:461, 1970.

CHAPTER 9

Radiation Therapy In The Management Of Breast Cancer

MYRON P. NOBLER

INTRODUCTION

For many decades radiation therapy has played an important part in the treatment of breast cancer. Clinical observation and data on radio-responsiveness indicate that most breast cancers are moderately radiosensitive and that long-term or permanent local control can be achieved by a variety of radiotherapeutic modalities and techniques. There are four distinctive situations in which irradiation may be employed: 1) for postoperative treatment, following a mastectomy; 2) as primary treatment of the breast cancer; 3) for preoperative treatment; and 4) for palliation of metastases and local recurrences.

Postoperative Irradiation

Radiation therapy has been employed following a mastectomy (total, modified radical, or radical) for many years. Although the term "prophylactic treatment" has been used, it is apparent that this is a misnomer. Radiation is beneficial only if it is therapeutic—i.e., if there are cancer cells present in the treatment field, their radiosensitivity and consequent death will ultimately improve local control rates. Irradiation can eradicate microscopic or subclinical disease that has spread beyond the margins of the surgical resection and thus reduce the incidence of local and regional recurrences. Irradiating an area where there are no cancer cells present will not prevent the appearance of metastatic cancer from occurring at any later time, often months or years following the radiation treatments. However, since it is not always possible to determine whether microscopic cancer is present in certain areas, the decision regarding radiation therapy must be made on the basis of probabilities. Thus, it is not always necessary for patients to receive postoperative irradiation. For example, the patient with a small tumor (under 2 cm) located in an outer quadrant, with no skin or muscle involvement, and with no axillary lymph node metastases, probably will not benefit from radiation therapy.

The purpose of postoperative irradiation of the chest wall and draining lymph node regions (internal mammary, axillary, and supraclavicular) is to improve permanent local control rates. By so doing, the quality of survival, if not the duration, may be improved. This has been demonstrated in many studies: Urban (1959) reported a 10% parasternal recurrence rate in 264 patients who did not have radiation therapy for central and inner quadrant tumors; Nelson and Montague (1975) reported *no* parasternal recurrences in 240 patients who had central and inner quadrant carcinomas and who *were* given postoperative irradiation to the internal mammary region. Fletcher (1972), and Nelson and Montague (1975) showed that if the axillary nodes are positive, then there will be supraclavicular recurrences in 20% to 26% of the patients if no postoperative radiation therapy is employed; whereas, with postoperative radiation therapy, this recurrence rate can be decreased to between 1.2% and 1.5%. Wallgren (1977) showed an overall local and regional recurrence rate involving the draining lymph nodes and the chest wall of approximately 28% in patients having only a mastectomy, versus 6% in a comparable group that received postoperative irradiation. Host and Brennhovd (1975), Nelson and Montague (1975), and Fletcher (1972) have analyzed other large groups of post-mastectomy patients and present additional statistical data showing local control rates that are comparable with those noted above and thus have substantiated further the indications for postoperative radiation therapy. In addition, our long-term results with postoperative irradiation at Beth Israel Hospital are also consistent with the above data.

One may also consider the impact of local radiation therapy upon overall survival rates; the argument has been posed that local irradaition will depress local anti-tumor (immunological?) mechanisms and may therefore result in decreased overall survival rates. This has been carefully examined by Order (1977), and McCredie (1976), and has not been substantiated. Rather, comparing surgical techniques alone with surgery combined with radiation therapy, the five- and 10-year survival figures are apparently better when radiation therapy is added.

Host and et al. (1977) studied a large number of patients with Stage II breast carcinoma with positive axillary lymph nodes that were randomized into two groups: One group had radical mastectomies followed by radiation therapy, and the other group had only radical mastectomies. The authors found that the sub-group that received postoperative irradaition had a five-year overall survival rate of 86%, while the sub-group that had only a radical mastectomy had a five-year survival of 70%. Chu et al. (1976) showed that postoperative radiation therapy given to a group of patients with moderately far advanced disease and positive metastasis to lymph nodes at the axillary apex resulted in a 39% survival, whereas a comparable group of patients not given radiation therapy had a 22% survival.

Data from the current Stockholm Trial (Einhorn, 1978) may be the most conclusive: Women with Stages I, II, and III breast carcinoma, randomized to have only a modified radical mastectomy, demonstrate a crude survival rate of 63%, compared with a matched group that received postoperative irradiation and has a 72% crude survival rate.

The most commonly performed mastectomy procedure at our hospital is a modified radical mastectomy, and, when we see potential candidates in consultation, our most commonly employed indications for postoperative radiation therapy are the following:

1) For a tumor less than 4 cm in size with no grave signs and no axillary lymph node metastases we do not advise postoperative irradaition if the tumor is located in an outer quadrant. But if this tumor is located medially or centrally, we irradiate the internal mammary lymph node chain.

2) For small tumors in any location, if there are only a few axillary lymph nodes containing metastatic disease (less then 20% of those removed), then we advise irradiating the lymph nodes in the internal mammary, the supraclavicular, and the axillary apex regions, but not the chest wall (Brady, et. al., 1977).

3)For large tumors (over 4 cm in size), or those presenting with one or more of the grave signs, we employ more extensive irradiation, which includes the entire chest wall, in addition to the draining lymph nodes in the internal mammary, supraclavicular, and axillary apex regions. The grave signs are: many positive metastases to axillary lymph nodes (over 20% of the nodes removed); carcinoma fixed to the pectoral fascia; carcinoma fixed to the skin; edema, *peau d' orange,* or erythema of the skin of the breast; a pathology report of multiple foci or carcinoma in the breast; a pathology report of vascular, lymphatic, or perineural invasion.

The above indications would also apply to the patient who has had a classical radical mastectomy. If the patient has had a total (simple) mastectomy for a small tumor without grave signs, we advise irradiation of the internal mammary, supraclavicular, and axillary lymph node regions. If a simple mastectomy was done for a tumor with one or more of the grave signs noted above, we advocate irradiation of the chest wall in addition to the regional lymph node groups.

The radiation treatments may be given with either an electron beam or more conventional megavoltage teletherapy, such as cobalt-60. If electron beam therapy is employed, the electron energy chosen will vary according to the area irradiated: thus, we would use a 6 MeV electron beam for the chest wall, a 9 MeV beam for the homolateral internal mammary lymph nodes, and a 12 MeV or 15 MeV electron beam for the supraclavicular region. Direct anterior portals are used to treat all these areas. If cobalt-60 teletherapy is employed, the chest wall and internal mammary lymph nodes are included in medial and lateral tangential portals (treatment tecnhiques are described in greater detail in the section below on primary radiation therapy of the breast). Also, when cobalt-60 is used to irradiate the supraclavicular-axillary apex region, we employ opposing anterior and posterior portals. The radiation dose delivered is 5000 rad, given over a period of five weeks, at a daily dose rate of 200 rad.

IRRADIATION AS THE PRIMARY TREATMENT FOR BREAST CARCINOMA

During the past decade radiation therapy has emerged as an acceptable alternative to mastectomy as the primary treatment for breast carcinoma. There are many women with operable and potentially curable localized breast cancer (Stage I or II) who cannot or will not undergo a mastectomy as primary treatment for a variety of reasons that fall into three general categories:

1) The women are considered to be inoperable because of serious medical problems or advanced age.

2) The women have serious psychiatric problems and are not considered suitable candidates for mastectomy.

3) There are women who want to retain their breasts, and, following a full discussion of the problem, choose irradiation over mastectomy; in some instances, women refuse a mastectomy despite a recommendation that it be performed in which case radiation therapy is then offered.

In this large group of women, it is obvious that every effort must be made to achieve permanent local control of the carcinoma, and this can be achieved in over 90% of the patients treated with local tumor excision or segmental resection of the breast, followed by total breast and lymph node irradiation.

There is another group of women, presenting with far advanced breast cancer (Stage III or IV), where mastectomy is contraindicated for the following reasons: extensive and unresectable local involvement; inflammatory carcinoma; documented distant metastases. In this latter advanced cancer group, there is still a fair chance for cure, enhanced if distant metastases do not develop. Therefore it is equally important for this group to achieve permanent local control of the breast carcinoma, and this again can be accomplished with aggressive, high dose, systematically employed supervoltage teletherapy.

This concept was initially established in a landmark paper (Peters, 1967). Peters has now followed the study group of 145 women with Stages I and II breast cancer for between five and 35 years and reports (Peters, 1975) a local control rate of 93% and a cumulative disease-free survival rate of 57%. Other more recently published studies, including our own series of patients, appears to be achieving similar results (Table I) in all stages, and it appears evident from these reports that local control rates with primary radiation therapy are comparable to those obtained with modified radical mastectomy and postoperative irradiation.

What remains to be determined is the impact of primary radiation therapy on long-term survival, compared to survival after surgery with or without irradiation. Peters' study was not prospective; rather, it was a retrospective analysis, creating matched pairs of cases treated either by biopsy plus radiation therapy (with a disease-free overall survival rate of 57%) or by mastectomy (radical or modified radical) plus irradiation (with a disease-free survival rate of 50%). The patients in the other published studies have not been followed long enough to determine true survival figures in comparison with surgical results, and they were not randomized. Therefore, we must await the results of a randomized prospective trial in order to determine conclusively whether there is an advantage to either modality. Of equal importance is the evaluation of the impact of either therapeutic modality on the appearance of distant metastases, since this is often the ultimate determining factor in survival. In Peters' (1977) report, which was again retrospective, the metastatic rate in the group that had mastectomies followed by irradiation was 24%, and in the group that had an excision biopsy followed by radiation therapy, the metastatic rate was only 12%.

In general, the diagnostic surgical procedures performed in patients who will be receiving primary radiation therapy are related to the stage of the carcinoma: Most Stage I and II patients will have either a segmental resection or an excision biopsy; in patients with more advanced disease, a generous incision biopsy usually will be done in order to obtain a sufficient amount of tissue to perform estrogen receptor studies.

The radiation therapy at our institution is planned as follows: The breast and adjacent chest wall tissues, including the mid- and lower-axillary lymph nodes and the internal mammary nodes, are irradiated via medial and lateral tangential portals. The lymph nodes in the axillary apex and the supraclavicular region are treated via opposing anterior and posterior portals. The upper margins of the tangential portals are matched to the lower

Table I.
Results of Primary Irradiation

Author	Stage	Number of Cases	Local Control Rate (%)	Cumulative N.E.D.* Survival Number of Cases	%	Number of Years Followed
Ghossein, et. al.	T-1 & T-2	36	94%	26/36	72%	2-9 yrs.
	T-3 & T-4	22	45%	4/22	18%	
Peters	I & II	145	93%	83/145	57%	5-35 yrs. (145 over 5 yrs.)
Prosnitz, et. al.	I & II	30	97%	26/30	87%	1-10 yrs. 27 under 5 yrs. 3 over 5 yrs.
Wallner, et. al.	I	20	85%	14/20	70%	0-14 yrs. 49 under 5 yrs. 2 over 5 yrs.
	II	2	50%	1/2	50%	
	III	28	89%	10/28	36%	
	IV	1	0	0	0	
Levene et. al.	I	19	100%	12/19	63%	2-8 yrs.
	II	45	100%	22/45	49%	
	III	86	68%	15/86	17%	
Spitalier, et. al.	T1-T2-No	152		130/152	85%	5-17 yrs.
	T1-T2-NI	144		102/144	71%	
	T3-No-NI	104		44/104	42%	
Beth Israel Series	I	20	100%	17/20	85%	1½-10 yrs. 77 under 5 yrs. 13 over 5 yrs.
	II	21	95%	10/21	48%	
	III	36	92%	12/36	33%	
	IV	13	100%	0/13	0%	

* N.E.D. = No evidence of active disease.

edges of the supraclavicular fields. The tangential portals are delineated by means of a clear plastic "breast box" that is rigidly attached to the head of the cobalt-60 unit. Tissue equivalent bolus is placed within the breast box in order to create a homogenous volume of irradiated tissue (chest wall, breast, tumor, skin and subcutaneous tissue, and draining lymph nodes) so that the dose distribution throughout the entire treated area is homogenous and equal. The bolus is usually withdrawn at a tumor dose of 3000 to 4000 rad when the patient has developed a significant erythematous skin reaction. The dose delivered to the entire breast is 6000 rad in most Stage I and II patients. If an extensive carcinoma was present initially, or if the tumor shows slow regression and residual disease is present at 6000 rad, then additional irradiation is given to increase the dose to 7000 rad, or else an iridium-192 interstitial implant is performed.

The supraclavicular and axillary regions receive a tumor dose of 5000 rad if clinically negative initially and 6000 rad if clinically positive at the outset. The dose is increased to 7000 rad or an implant is performed if indicated to control residual tumor. A modified "split course" of treatment is almost always employed: When the skin reactions reach their peak, treatments are temporarily discontinued for one or two weeks. Thus, the total tumor dose of 6000 to 7000 rad is usually delivered over a period of seven to nine weeks.

Side effects and complications of treatment are minimal. During treatment an acute erythematous skin reaction always develops. This is caused by the bolus and is necessary as an indication that the skin has received a full tumor dose. The skin reaction is treated symptomatically with aquafor ointment and will subside spontaneously. Some patients will report mild pharyngitis or esophagitis; this can be treated symptomatically and will subside after treatments have been concluded. Other acute side effects may occur during treatment, and have been reported in the literature, but we have not observed any clinical, laboratory, or x-ray evidence to suggest acute carditis, pleuritis, pneumonitis, mediastinitis, or pericarditis.

We have seen edema of the breast as a common subacute reaction, causing temporary discomfort. This occasionally progressed to a mild chronic breast edema, which was neither painful nor disabling. Rarely, a mild degree of chronic breast fibrosis or axillary fibrosis occured. One of our patients developed two rib fractures in a heavily irradiated axillary region. Serial chest x-rays will often demonstrate the late appearance of apical pulmonary fibrosis and thickening of the pleura on the anterior chest wall. However, radiation pnemonitis and radiation-induced pulmonary fibrosis have not been evident radiographically elsewhere in the lungs and, in our experience, have not been clinically evident as a late complication of irradiation.

The evaluation of cosmetic results is extremely important, especially in the group of women who refused mastectomy because of the desire to retain the breast. These women were consistently satisfied with the final results. Generally, these patients received a total breast radiation dosage of approximately 6000 rad. The side effects and long-range chronic effects noted above occurred primarily in those patients in whom the initial presence of disease was more extensive and for whom the dose delivered to the entire breast was usually in the range of 6500 to 7000 rad. Other chronic skin radiation effects were noted, primarily in those patients who received doses in excess of 6000 rad. These effects included subcutaneous fibrosis, atrophy of the dermis and epidermis, and the appearance of telangiectasia. The cosmetic results in these patients was, understandably, somewhat less than perfect, but since the desired goal of permanent local control was achieved, the cosmetic effects were considered acceptable by both the patients and their physicians (Fig. 1).

In our potentially curable Stage I and II cases treated only with irradiation, we have been able to achieve local results that are comparable to those obtained with modified radical mastectomy and postoperative radiation

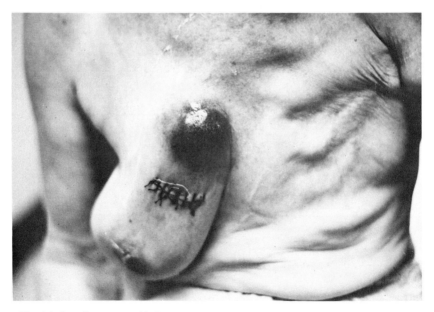

Fig. 1A. Locally unresectable breast cancer with ulceration, fixation to chest wall, and multiple staellite nodules.

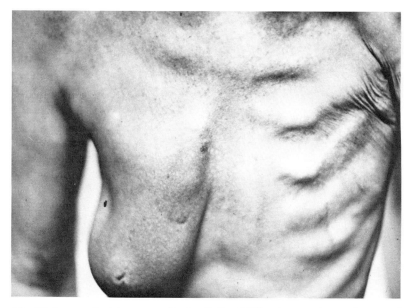

Fig. 1B. Same patient two years after irradiation (6000 rad tumor dose to breast and draining lymph node regions delivered in eight weeks.)

therapy (Table I). Furthermore, many of these women with tenuous medical conditions have been spared the risks of general anesthesia and major surgery, and those women with a strong desire to retain their breasts have been able to do so safely. At the least, in these cases, irradiation can improve the quality of survival and does not appear to be detrimental to the duration of survival.

It is apparent that the majority of our patients with Stage III cancers will develop clinical evidence of disseminated metastases within a period of six to 18 months after diagnosis and initial treatment. Therefore, it is extremely beneficial to these patients to be able to achieve permanent or long-term local control of a massive, ulcerating, fungating, infected, painful breast carcinoma with irradiation, thereby obviating an extensive surgical procedure and probable postoperative radiation therapy. In our Stage IV patients initially presenting with documented distant metastases, we have noted an average period of survival of over 24 months when the patients are treated comprehensively with multiple therapeutic modalities. Thus, it is equally essential to provide permanent or long-term local control of the usually-extensive local cancers, again eliminating the necessity of performing major surgery. Therefore, by establishing local control of the breast carcinoma in advanced Stage III and IV cases, as demonstrated by our own results and those in other reported series (Table I), we can improve the quality of the patients' survival time as well as contribute to their overall longevity.

PREOPERATIVE RADIATION THERAPY

There are a number of therapeutic advantages that can be derived from preoperative irradiation. These relate to the destruction of cancer cells by the high energy gamma rays or x-rays, resulting in shrinkage of the tumor, with consequent conversion of an unresectable carcinoma to a resectable one. Even if the carcinoma cells are not totally destroyed, the radiation effect is still manifest, since damaged carcinoma cells will not be able to metabolize normally and, therefore, will not be able to grow or replicate. Thus, theoretically, there will be a great decrease in local recurrences and, for those cancer cells that do escape into the blood stream or lymphatics at the time of surgical manipulation, there will be a lesser likelihood of these cells implanting at distant sites and forming the nidus for later development of clinical metastatic disease. Preoperative radiation therapy has been most successfully employed in adenocarcinoma of the endometrium, carcinoma of the bladder, adenocarcinoma of the rectosigmoid colon, and a wide variety of epidermoid carcinomas of the head and neck region, and is commonly utilized in all these areas almost routinely.

In our own experience, preoperative irradiation in treatment of breast cancer has been useful, but the technique has been employed relatively infrequently. Despite the fact that a significant retrospective study done by Fletcher in 1967 showed a 10% improvement in survival rates when preoperative radiation therapy was used, it was not until 1970 that a controlled prospective trail was mounted. In the Stockholm breast cancer trail (Wallgren, 1977, and Einhorn, 1978) 960 patients, all under 70 years of age and all with operable breast carcinoma (Stages I, II or III), were included in the study and divided by randomization into three groups of equal size—no radiation therapy, preoperative radiation therapy, and postoperative irradiation. A modified radical mastectomy was performed on all patients. The preoperative radiation therapy techniques employed were identical with the tecnhiques described above in this chapter for total breast radiation therapy, but the doses were lower (4500 rad in five weeks). Surgery was done six weeks after completion of irradiation.

The 960 patients have all been followed for a minimum of two, and up to seven years (360 patients have now been followed for over five years). The overall survival rate in the group receiving preoperative radiation therapy is 77%, in the group receiving postoperative irradiation 72%; the group of patients having only a modified radical mastectomy has a 63% overall survival rate. Local recurrence rates in the group receiving either preoperative or postoperative irradiation are approximately 6%, whereas in group with the radical mastectomy only, approximately 28% developed local recurrences. When the groups are analyzed according to tumor size, location, axillary lymph node involvement, age, pre- or postmenopausal stage, or any other criteria, the statistics are unchanged, and it is still evident that the preoperative irradiation group demonstrates the best overall results, and the group having only surgery demonstrates the poorest overall results.

The advantages of preoperative radiation therapy have been summarized above. The disadvantages are a slightly higher incidence of delayed wound healing and of local surgical complications, and a slightly higher incidence of arm edema. If the long-range advantages continue to outweigh the disadvantages, then preoperative radiation therapy will undoubtedly become a technique that will be utilized much more frequently in the future.

PALLIATIVE IRRADIATION

Notwithstanding the tremendous strides made in recent years in chemotherapy and hormonal manipulation of metastatic breast cancer, local palliative irradiation still represents the most rapid, most effective, and most efficient means of achieving palliation for metastatic lesions in most situations, and also of treating local recurrences.

Skeletal metastases are commonly seen and may involve any bone in the body. Pain is the most common and most disabling symptom, as the metastatic carcinoma expands and destroys normal bone. Pathological fractures may develop with minimal or no trauma. The following dose schedule will usually achieve local stabilization with local destruction of the carcinoma, allowing the bones to heal, and relieving pain: In a limited treatment area (i.e., a portion of an extremity) we can give relatively high doses in a short period of time (400 to 500 rad daily for one week) for a high therapeutic efficiency. If a larger area is involved (especially multiple vertebral bodies), daily doses can not exceed 200 to 300 rad without producing the symptoms of some side effects of irradiation, and the treatment course must be spread out over a longer period of time. Thus, 3000 rad delivered in two weeks (and up to 3,500 rad in three weeks) is the usual dose.

With more extensive disease, producing compression fractures of the spinal cord, we must irradiate early and aggressively to forestall the growth of the carcinoma into the spinal canal, which may result in spinal cord compression and paraplegia. In the presence of pathological fractures of the extremities, we have found that it is often very effective to obtain orthopedic fixation of the involved bone first, and then give postoperative radiation therapy up to a dose of 3000 to 3500 rad in three weeks.

Hematogenous metastases to organs are also quite common in advanced breast carcinoma, and radiation therapy is equally effective here. A dose level of 3000 rad in three weeks is usually the minimum dose needed to control soft tissue or organ metastases, although occasionally this may have to be increased to 4000 rad in four weeks. Liver metastases can be successfully irradiated by a dose of 3000 rad in four weeks without significantly destroying whatever remains of normal liver function. Local soft tissue tumor metastases to the epigastric region or pelvis can be treated in a similar fashion. Pulmonary metastases can also be irradiated, but the field must be small (less than one half of the lung volume) or else radiation pneumonitis may develop and itself become a serious management problem.

Brain metastases unfortunately occur frequently in metastatic breast cancer. These can be treated by combined corticosteroid therapy and irradiation. Normal brain tissue is generally quite radioresistant. Therefore we can deliver a tumor dose of 3000 rad in two weeks, or up to 4000 rads in four weeks to the entire brain, and achieve excellent local palliation.

Finally, local chest wall and draining lymph node recurrences represent one of the major therapeutic problems we face. Often, these local recurrences are the only evidence of active carcinoma, and can be quite indolent, growing slowly over a long period of time. It is therefore extremely important to achieve control of these lesions. Generally they can be effectively controlled by a wide variety of radiotherapeutic techniques, including external therapy with cobalt-60, Linear Accelerators, or electron beams, and implants with iridium-192 or other radionuclides. Doses necessary to control these lesions are generally in the range of 4000 to 6000 rad in four to six weeks and can be achieved without difficulty. The specific techniques employed are similar to those described in earlier sections of this chapter on giving radiation therapy with curative intent, although the time-dose relationships may vary somewhat. The eventual result, however, is usually excellent long-term local control.

REFERENCES

Brady, L., Fletcher, G., Levitt, S. Cancer of the breast: the role of radiation therapy after mastectomy. *Cancer* 39:2868, 1977.

Chu, F.C., Lucas, J.C., Farrow, J.H., Nickson, J.J. Does prophylactic radiotherapy given for cancer of the breast predispose to metastasis? *Amer. Jnl. Roentgenol.* 99:987, 1976.

Einhorn, J. Adjuvant radiotherapy in operable breast cancer: the results of the Stockholm trial. Presented at the 60th annual meeting of The American Radium Society. New Orleans, April, 1978.

Fletcher, G.H. The advantages of preoperative irradiation. *J.A.M.A.* 200:140, 1967.

Fletcher, G.H. Local results of irradiation in the primary management of localized breast cancer. *Cancer* 29: 545, 1972.

Ghossein, N., Stacey, P., Alpert, S., Ager, P., Krishnaswamey, V. Local control of breast cancer with tumorectomy plus radiotherapy or radiotherapy alone. *Radiology* 121: 455, 1976.

Host, H., Brennhovd, I.O. Combined surgery and radiation therapy versus surgery alone in primary mammary carcinoma. *Acta Radiol., Ther., Phys, and Biol.* 14: 25, 1975.

Host, H., Brennhovd, I.O. The effect of postoperative radiotherapy in breast cancer. *Int. Jnl. Rad. Oncol., Biol, and Phys.* 2: 1061, 1977.

Levene, M., Harris, J., Hellman, S. Treatment of carcinoma of the breast by radiation therapy. *Cancer* 39: 2840, 1977.

Mc Credie, J.A., Immunologic considerations of large volume radiotherapy. *Jnl. Can. Assoc. Radiol.* 27: 264, 1976.

Nelson, A.J., Montague, E.D. Management of localized carcinoma of the breast. *J.A.M.A.* 231: 189, 1975.

Nobler, M.P., Venet, L. Unpublished data.

Order, S. Beneficial and detrimental effects of therapy on immunity in breast cancer. *Int. Jnl. Rad. Oncol., Biol., & Phys.* 2: 377, 1977.

Peters, M.V. Wedge resection and irradiation - an effective treatment in early breast cancer. *J.A.M.A.* 200: 144, 1967.

Peters, M.V. Cutting the "Gordian knot" in early breast cancer. *Annals of The Royal College of Physicians and Surgeons of Canada.* 8: 186, 1975.

Peters, M.V., Wedge resection with or without radiation in early breast cancer. *Int. Jnl. Rad. Oncol, Biol., & Phys.* 2:1151, 1977.

Prosnitz, L., Goldenberg, I. Radiation therapy as primary treatment for early stage carcinoma of the breast. *Cancer* 35: 1587, 1975.

Spitalier, J., Brandone, H., Ayme, Y., Amalric, R., Santamaria, F., & Seigle, J. Cesium therapy of breast cancer: a five year report on 400 consecutive patients. *Int. Jnl. Rad. Oncol, Biol, & Phys.* 2:231, 1977.

Urban, J.A. Clinical experience and results of excision of the internal mammary lymph node chain in primary operable breast cancer. *Cancer* 12: 14, 1959.

Wallgren, A. A controlled study: preoperative versus postoperative irradiation. *Int. J Rad. Oncol. Biol, & Phys.* 2: 1167, 1977.

Wallner, P., Brady, L., Loughead, J., Matsumoto, T., Antoniades, J., Prasasvinichai, S., Glassburn, J., Asbell, S., Damsker, J. Subtotal mastectomy and radiation therapy in the definitive management of localized breast malignancy. *Am. J. Roentgenol.* 127:505, 1976.

CHAPTER 10

Reconstruction Of The Breast After Mastectomy

SAUL HOFFMAN

Loss of a breast is a traumatic experience for even the most well-adjusted woman. Post-mastectomy depression, which is marked by anxiety, insomnia, thoughts of suicide and feelings of shame and worthlessness, is common (Renneker et al., 1952). Physicans are becoming more aware of these important psychological aspects. In addition, post-mastectomy deformities are no longer acceptable to many women who are seeking restoration of body image. Recognition of the need for rehabilitation after mastectomy and the trend to less radical surgery have led to increasing interest in breast reconstuction.

HISTORY

Attempts to reconstruct the breast after mastectomy can be traced back to the last century, when Verneuil (1887) used a portion of the healthy breast to replace the missing one. Since then, there have been many reports describing the use of part or all of the remaining breast for this purpose. Kleinschmidt (1924) described a procedure in which a thoraco-abdominal flap, adjacent to the mammary defect, was used to create a new breast. From that time to the present, a variety of local flaps have been described, modified, forgotten, and then reintroduced to resurface defects of the chest wall and reconstruct the breasts after mastectomy.

Sir Harold Gillies (1945) brought skin and subcutaneous tissue from the mid-abdomen to the chest by means of a tube pedicle. The umbilicus was included and everted to stimulate a nipple. After that, various abdominal and chest flaps were attempted.

Earlier, Czerny (1895) transplanted a lipoma from a patient's back to her breast to repair a defect resulting from removal of a fibroadenoma. This was probably the first breast reconstruction using a free graft. Attempts to replace missing breast tissue with free grafts of fat, fat-fascia, and dermal fat have been abandoned because of the high rate of absorption.

Cronin and Gerow (1963) developed a silicone prosthesis for use in breast augmentation. Snyderman and Guthrie (1971) tried the silicone implant for breast reconstruction after mastectomy and presented their experiences in 1971. The resulting appearances of their early patients was unsatisfactory. With improvement in surgical techniques and in types of prostheses and with the trend to less radical surgery for breast cancer, more acceptable results have been obtained.

CASE SELECTION OF CANDIDATES

Ideally, the plastic surgeon should see the patient prior to mastectomy, in order to select, with her participation, the type of incision to be used and to decide if nipple banking is advisable. A preoperative consultation will also alleviate the anxieties of many women who will be relieved to learn that breast reconstruction is available.

In some situations, immediate reconstruction can be considered. This has been done at the time of the mastectomy or several days later (Hueston et al., 1970). It is generally wise, however, to wait until induration has subsided and the skin is mobile over the chest wall. This may take anywhere from three to twelve months.

The details of the operation, limitations, and possible complications are carefully explained. Patients with unrealistic expectations or severe emotional problems are seen several times preoperatively and referred to a psychiatrist when necessary, before a decision regarding surgery is made.

Contraindications

Reconstruction is mainly contraindicated for the patient with unrealistic expectations who will be unhappy, even with good surgical results. It may be helpful to show patients photographs to help explain the procedure and its limitations. The tempatation to show only the best results should be avoided.

The presence of metastases is probably a contraindication to reconstruction. Outright refusal to perform reconstruction, however, may have a devastating effect on a young woman who is hoping her disease will be cured. She should be told that reconstruction may be possible, but that it should be postponed until she has been off chemotherapy for several months. In this way, all hope will not be denied. There is no evidence tbat reconstruction speeds up the disease process. In rare circumstances, therefore, it might be considered worthwhile for emotional support. Since recent evidence indicates that most chemotherapeutic agents do not interfere significantly with wound healing, some surgeons will begin reconstruction while the patient is on chemotherapy (Cohen et al., 1975). Most, however, prefer to delay surgery until after the treatment has been discontinued.

While reconstruction is not contraindicated after radical surgery, it is more difficult. Several stages are required to replace the thin, scarred skin which will not tolerate an implant. This also holds true when the skin has been damaged by radiotherapy. Some women are not willing to accept the limitations or to undergo the additional surgery necessary for reconstruction in these cases.

TECHNIQUE

The operation begins with preoperative planning. Since it is difficult to determine the proper position for the implant with the patient on the operating table, it should be done in advance with the patient seated. Because the inframammary fold will move upward upon insertion of the prosthesis, it is placed 1 cm to 2 cm below the normal side. The new fold and the extent of undermining is marked with a 20% solution of silver nitrate. The marks will remain for several days. After bilateral mastectomies, planning is aided by having the patient wear her brassiere and external prostheses.

A mid-axillary vertical incision, 8 cm to 10 cm in length is made and carried forward to the border of the pectoralis muscle (Fig. 1a). The subpectoral plane is entered and a pocket dissected large enough to allow some movement of the prosthesis (Fig. 1b). A retractor with a fiberoptic light source facilitates the dissection and hemostasis, which is obtained with an electrocoagulator. When there is adequate residual skin and subcutaneous tissue, the prosthesis can be placed subcutaneously, as in routine augmentation mammoplasty. The posterior skin flap is undermined and advanced anteriorly to close the vertical relaxing incision. A catheter attached to suction will help prevent fluid accumulation postoperatively (Fig. 1c).

There are several variations, depending on the type of case and the preference of the surgeon, as described below.

Placement of the Incision

The mid-axillary vertical incision relaxes the pectoral skin, allowing it to be mobilized anteriorly. It also has the advantage of not overlying the im-

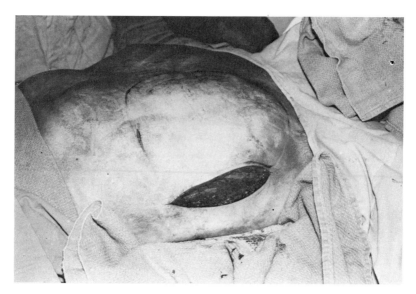

Fig. 1a. Incision is carried forward to the border of the pectoralis muscle. Note relaxation obtained by anterior advancement of skin flap. Preoperative markings outline extent of undermining and inframammary fold.

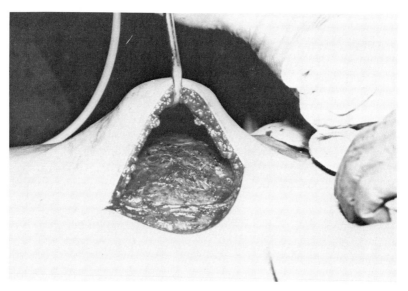

Fig. 1b. Completion of dissection is facilitated by the use of a fiberoptic retractor. Note the large subpectoral pocket obtained by wide undermining.

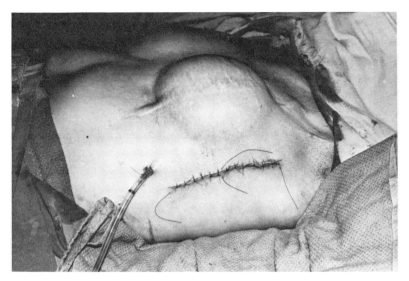

Fig. 1c. Patient is shown after insertion of the prosthesis and wound closure. Note presence of suction catheter.

plant. The main disadvantage of this incision is the difficulty of exposing the inferior and medial portion of the pocket.

A transverse, inframammary incision provides easier access for the dissection and can be placed to stimulate the inframammary fold. It may, however, interfere with the vertically oriented blood supply to the pectoral skin.

Occasionally, an additional scar can be avoided by reopening the lateral portion of a transverse mastectomy incision to insert the prosthesis. It is also possible to utilize the original mastectomy incision, undermine widely, and place the implant without creating an additional scar (Birnbaum et al., 1978). With this method, the implant must be anchored in order to prevent skin compromise with this technique, the implant can be partially inflated, adding more saline after the wound has healed.

Type of Prosthesis

Breast prostheses are made from silicone, a synthetic material which is very well tolerated by the body. There has been no clinical or experimental evidence of tumor formation or other deleterious effects with this substance (Lilla et al., 1976). There is a tendency, however, for a fibrous capsule to form around the implant which can cause pressure and excessive firmness (Imber et al., 1974).

One type of implant is a contoured silicone bag inflated with saline. The volume can be adjusted during the operation and supplemented as skin stretches later on. In another type of implant, the silicone bag is filled with silicone gel, which has a consistency similar to that of breast tissue and is available in various shapes and sizes. Some surgeons prefer a prosthesis that is divided into three compartments by a Y-shaped internal membrane; advocates of this implant claim it allows for a better contour (Guthrie, 1976). A thin polyurethane covering allows for fixation to the surrounding tissue. This can be a disadvantage, since there may be some tissue reaction and removal of the implant is more difficult (Imber et al., 1974; Cocke et al., 1975).

While there is a wide variety of prostheses available, special problems may necessitate the use of a custom-made implant (Figs. 2a-2c). These may be inflatable, constructed with gel, or may incorporate inflatability and gel. Since the contour is largely determined by the tightness of the overlying skin, it is doubtful that the problem of contour can be completely solved by a more ideal implant. One approach has been to stretch the skin with an implant, which is gradually inflated over a period of time, and then to insert a custom-made prosthesis.

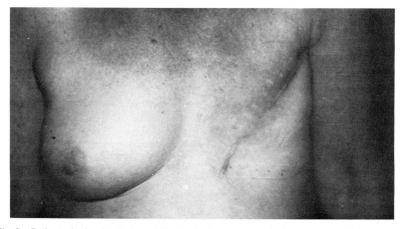

Fig. 2a. Patient who has had left modified radical mastectomy is shown one year after surgery.

Residual subclavicular depression after a radical mastectomy is more disturbing than is the loss of the breast to many women, since the deformity is

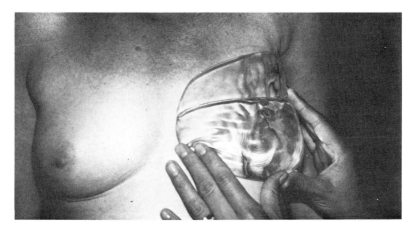

Fig. 2b. Custom-made dual compartment silicone gel implant, was created from a moulage of the normal breast.

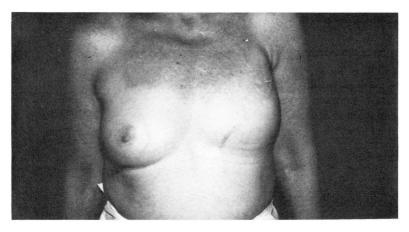

Fig. 2c. Patient is shown one year post reconstruction, does not want nipple reconstruction.

not easily hidden by most clothing. A custom-made implant sometimes can correct this problem, but the results have been disappointing and an exact fit is almost impossible to accomplish.

RECONSTRUCTION AFTER RADICAL MASTECTOMY

If the patient is highly motivated and will acecept the limitations and additional risks, there are several methods available. A flap of skin and subcutaneous tissue can be obtained from the upper abdomen or lower chest and used to replace damaged pectoral skin (Cronin et al., 1977). The flap is oriented transversely and based medially, receiving its blood supply from the thoraco-epigastric vessels. It is rotated 90 degrees into a vertical direction and inset into the defect. By staging, the flap can be made long enough to correct a subclavicular depression. The donor site is closed primarily, except in extremely thin patients in whom a skin graft may be needed.

Reconstruction with an abdominal tube pedicle continues to be performed by some surgeons, often with acceptable results (Millard, 1976). A tube of excess abdominal skin and subcutaneous tissue is created and transferred to the chest in several stages. Here it may be used to resurface the chest wall and create a new breast. If further augmentation is required, a silicone implant is then inserted under this flap. This method has had rather limited application because of the number of stages and the considerable scarring produced.

The latissimus dorsi musculocutaneous flap has recently been described for breast reconstruction and appears to have considerable promise (McGraw et al., 1977). The principle of this flap is based on the fact that skin overlying a muscle receives a good deal of its blood supply from that muscle. It can, therefore, be moved as a unit as long as it remains attached at its dominant vascular pedicle. This allows a large defect to be resurfaced with well vascularized skin and muscle. After a radical mastectomy, the pectoralis muscle is absent and the skin flaps are likely to be thin and tight. In these cases, the latissimus dorsi muscle, together with an island of overlying skin, is moved from the back to the chest in one stage. A prosthesis is then placed under the muscle. There will, of course, be a residual scar on the back and the loss of muscle function may be of concern to some patients. It is of interest to note that in 1912, d'Este[18] described a flap of skin and latissimus dorsi muscle to repair a defect of the anterior chest wall (d'Este, 1912).

The omentum has been used to replace missing breast tissue after mastectomy or as a protective cover for an implant (Arnold, et al., 1976). It is very vascular and will even support a skin graft over a prosthesis. The omentum has also been used successfully in chest wall reconstruction (Jacobs et al., 1976). Of course, a laparotomy is necessary.

In most instances, the reconstructed breast will not match the remaining breast in size or contour, and further surgery must be done. This may consist of a mastopexy, a tightening up of the sagging skin. The nipple must also be relocated so that its position relative to the breast is appropriate. A reduction in breast size may be necessary. It is at this time that the nipple is reconstructed.

NIPPLE RECONSTRUCTION

Several techniques are available for nipple reconstruction. When the remaining nipple and areola are large enough, they can provide material for the new nipple: The peripheral portion of the areola can be used; the entire nipple can be removed as a full thickness skin graft and divided into two; or a split thickness skin graft of nipple and areola may be taken. If there is a lack of sufficient material, the labia will provide tissue of similar color and consistency. Free grafts from other areas or tattooing have also been recommended. In order to build up the central nipple projection, dermal, cartilage or onlay labial grafts have been recommended.

Nipple Banking

In order to facilitate reconstruction, the nipple may be removed from the specimen at the time of the mastectomy and replaced as a full thickness graft in the groin or thigh (Millard et al., 1971) (Fig. 3). It can subsequently be replaced on the reconstructed breast. Since the nipple comes from a breast that contains malignancy, there has been considerable debate about the advisability of this procedure (Smith et al., 1976). It is generally felt,

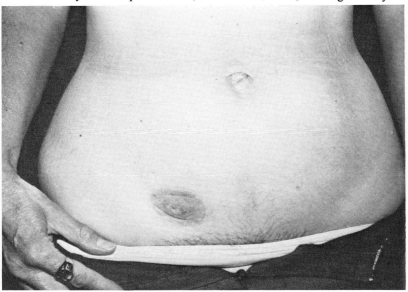

Fig. 3. Patient with a banked nipple.

however, that nipple banking is safe when the tumor is small and far enough away from the nipple. In addition, tissue from under the nipple must be examined and found free of pathology, and the ducts should be completely excised.

Technique

A partial thickness circle of skin is removed above the inguinal ligament into which the nipple areolar complex is sutured as a full thickness graft. If two nipples will be needed and the areolar is large enough, it can be divided and placed on two recipient sites. At the second stage, the nipple is removed again as a full thickness skin graft, making it slightly thinner to remove the subdermal scar and placing it on a de-epithelialized circle of skin on the reconstructed breast. (The position of the nipple should be marked out before surgery with the patient seated.) An elipse that includes the donor site is then removed and closed in a straight line. This leaves a small transverse lower abdominal scar, which is usually quite inconspicuous. Figures 4a to 4d show patient who has had nipple reconstruction and mastopexy.

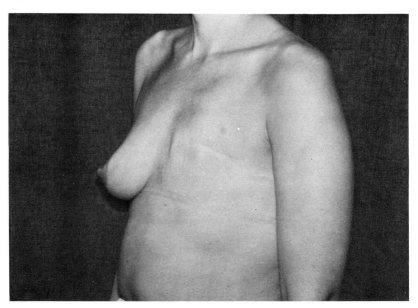

Fig. 4a. A 35-year-old woman after a right modified radical mastectomy. Left breast is slightly ptotic.

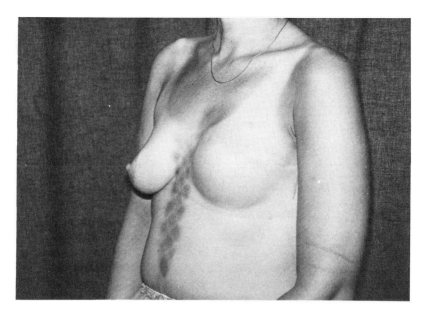

Fig. 4b. Appearance three months after placement of an inflatable silicone prosthesis under the pectoral muscle.

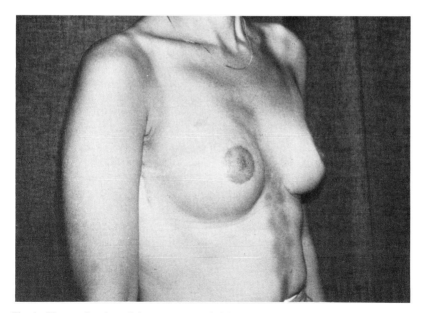

Fig. 4c. Six months after a left mastopexy and right nipple reconstruction. The excess areola and nipple were taken from the left breast.

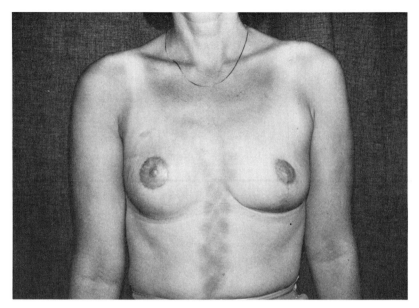

Fig. 4d. Front view of the same patient.

MANAGEMENT OF THE CONTRALATERAL BREAST

We have already discussed surgery on the contralateral breast for cosmetic reasons. A mastopexy or reduction mammoplasty is performed to create symmetry with the reconstructed breast (Figs. 4c and 4d). There are patients, however, in whom it is advisable to perform a total mastectomy for prophylaxis on the contralateral breast for example, in women who have an increased risk of developing cancer in the second breast (i.e., very young women, patients with multinodular breasts in which several biopsies have already been performed, and/or women with a strong family history of breast cancer).

In these cases, a total mastectomy with simultaneous reconstruction is recommended. When the pathology is in doubt or primary skin closure difficult, the implant can be inserted in a subsequent operation and the nipple banked. The results of reconstruction in these cases are generally satisfactory, since the remaining skin flaps are thick and have good circulation. Total mastectomy with conservative skin removal and replacement of the nipple will also allow for satisfactory reconstruction since there is adequate skin as well as muscle to protect the silicone implant.

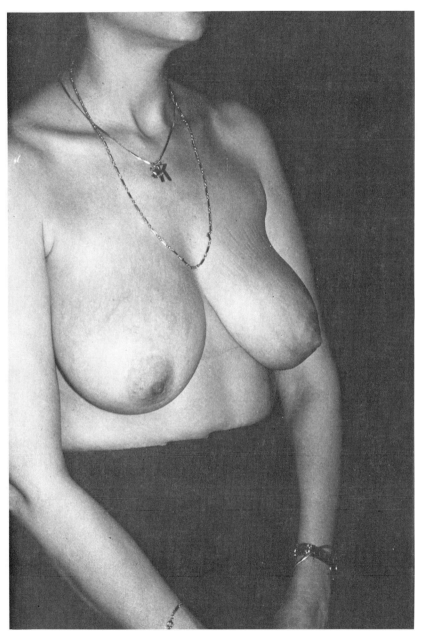

Fig. 5a. A 35-year-old woman with large, ptotic, multinodular breasts. Examination was difficult and there were two previous biopsies.

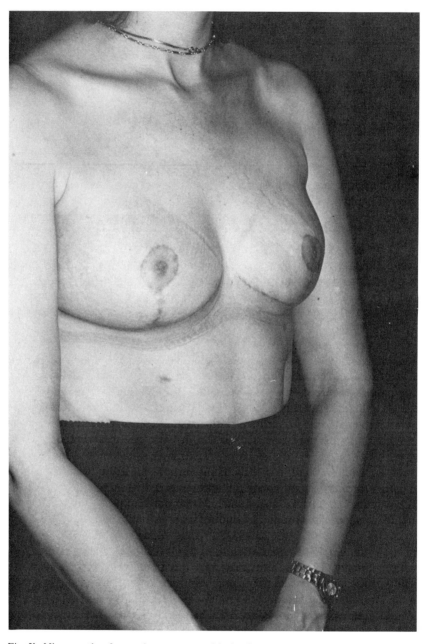

Fig. 5b. Nine months after total mastectomy with simultaneous reconstruction, using silicone gel implants.

Subcutaneous mastectomy has been advocated as a prophylactic treatment for breast cancer (Pennisi et al., 1971; Fredricks, 1975). It has also been suggested as a definitive procedure for certain small breast cancers (Freeman, 1973). Whether there is a place for this operation in the prophylaxis or treatment of cancer at all, is controversial (Hutter et al. 1973; Synderman, 1974; Peacock, 1975).

The technique of subcutaneous mastectomy was first described in 1917 by Bartlet (Bartlet, 1917). An inframammary incision was made through which the breast tissue was removed. Reconstruction was performed with free grafts of fat. The high rate of absorption of free fat grafts prompted a search for a satisfactory prosthetic material to replace the breast tissue. Silicone has been the best synthetic thus far, but there are still problems associated with its use.

More recently, Freeman described his technique (1962). Reconstruction was immediate or delayed, depending on the size of the breast and the resulting defect. He stated that many of the implants became firm and contracted, but at that time polyurethane prostheses were being used. Since then, the prostheses have improved, but capsular contracture is still a problem.

It is generally agreed that all of the breast tissue cannot be removed with this operation (Goldman et al., 1973). Techniques that remove the nipple and subareolar tissue and replace it as a full thickness graft do allow for a more thorough excision and can be applied to the larger, ptotic breast (Horton, 1974; Spira, 1977). Skin and nipple losses are less common with these methods and the esthetic results are superior.

COMPLICATIONS OF RECONSTRUCTION

At a recent meeting, the results of a survey on breast reconstruction were presented (Cocke et al., 1975). Of 1,536 plastic surgeons, 359 had performed 1,186 reconstructions following mastectomy for cancer. The incidence of complications was surprisingly low, and about 88% of the patients were pleased with the results. Perhaps it is still too early to determine the incidence of complications, since skin breakdown over the implant has been reported up to 10 years post-reconstruction (Hartwell et al., 1976). The following complications have been encountered:

Capsular Contracture

This can occur around a prosthesis even after augmentation mammoplasty. When it does, the implant becomes distorted, firm, and sometimes painful. Reoperation with release of the contracture may be necessary, but recurrence is common. Daily mobilization of the implant to maintain a slightly larger pocket has been helpful in preventing this problem.

Displacement of the Implant

This complication may occur if the pocket is dissected too far laterally or inferiorly. An inferior displacement can often be managed conservatively, however, by strapping the implant in the proper position. Superior displacement is more common and can usually be avoided by applying daily pressure in a downward direction to maintain the inferior sulcus. In these cases, reoperation may be necessary to reposition the implant.

Infection

When an infection occurs in the presence of a large implant, treatment is difficult without removing the prosthesis. Prophylactic antibiotics are thought to be of some value in preventing infection in these cases. Antibiotics have proven to be most effective when started preoperatively.

Loss of Implant

This complication generally occurs with severe capsular contracture. The skin overlying the prosthesis gradually becomes thin and atrophic, with subsequent exposure necessitating removal of the implant. It may be possible to replace the attenuated skin with a pedicle flap and subsequently replace the implant.

THE FUTURE OF BREAST RECONSTRUCTION

Earlier diagnosis, coupled with less radical surgery for breast cancer will provide more suitable candidates for reconstruction. As the procedure becomes more accepted by general surgeons, it will be offered to more women, just as reconstruction is offered for ablation of any other body part after cancer surgery.

As surgical techniques improve, it may be possible to reconstruct the breast routinely at the time of the mastectomy. A similar evolution took place in the management of head and neck cancer.

Microvascular surgery now allows the transfer of large amounts of tissue from one part of the body to another in a single stage (Fujino et al., 1975). This may facilitate replacement of skin and muscle after radical surgery, so that reconstruction can be done in one or two stages, if not immediately.

The plastic surgeon is now a permanent member of the team that manages patients with breast cancer. Perhaps one day mastectomy will no longer be necessary. Until that time, however, we must continue our efforts to improve the results of surgical rehabilitation of mastectomy patients.

REFERENCES

Arnold, P.G., Hartrampf, C.R., Jurkiewicz, M.J. One-stage reconstruction of the breast using transposed greater omentum. *Plast. & Reconst. Surg.* 57:520, 1976.

Bartlett, W. Anatomic substitute for the female breast. *Ann. Sug.* 66:208, 1917.

Birnbaum, L., Olsen, J.A. Breast reconstruction following radical mastectomy, using custom designed implants. *Plast. & Reconst. Surg.* 61:355, 1978.

Cocke, W.M., Leathers, H.K., Lynch, J.B. Foreign body reactions to polyurethane covers of some breast prostheses. *Plast. & Reconst. Sug.* 56:527, 1975.

Cocke, W.M., Lynch, J.B. Number and type of breast reconstructions done after radical mastectomy: Results of a survey of the society. Presented at the meeting of the American Society of Plastic and Reconstructive Surgeons. Toronto, Oct. 21, 1975.

Cohen, S.C., Gabelnick, H.L., Johnson, R.K., Golding, A. Effects of antineoplastic agents on wound healing in mice. *Surgery* 78:238, 1975.

Cronin, T., Gerow, F.J. Augmentation mammoplasty: a new "natural feel" prosthesis. In Transactions of the Third International Congress of Plastic Surgery. Exerpta Medica Foundation, Amsterdam, 1963.

Cronin, T.D., Upton, J., McDonough, J.M. Reconstruction of the breast after mastectomy. *Plast. & Reconst. Sug.* 59:1, 1977.

Czerny, V. Plasticher Ersatz der Brustdrüse durch ein Lipom. *Zentralbl. f. Chir.* 27:72, 1895.

d'Este, S.: La technique de l'amputation de la mamelle par le procédé de Tansini et sur une nouvelle application de cette operation; étude anatomo-clinique et operatoire. *Rev. Chir.* (Paris) 14:164, 1912.

Fredricks, S. A 10-year experience with subcutaneous mastectomy. *Clinics in Plast. Surg.* 2:347, 1975.

Freeman, B.S. Subcutaneous mastectomy for central tumors of the breast with immediate reconstruction. *Plast. & Reconst. Surg.* 51:263, 1973.

Freeman, B.S. Subcutaneous mastectomy for benign breast lesions with immediate or delayed prosthetic replacement. *Plast. & Reconst. Surg.* 30:676, 1962.

Fujino, T., Harashina, T., Aoyagi, F. Reconstruction for aplasia of the breast and pectoral region by microvascular transfer of a free flap from the buttock. *Plast. & Reconst. Sug.* 56:178, 1975.

Gillies, H. Operative replacement of the mammary prominence. *Brit. J. Surg.* 32:477, 1945.

Goldman, L.D., Goldwyn, R.M. Some anatomical considerations of subcutaneous mastectomy. *Plast. & Reconst. Surg.* 51:501, 1973.

Guthrie, R.H. Breast reconstruction after radical mastectomy. *Plast. & Reconst. Surg.* 57:14, 1976.

Hartwell, S.W., Anderson, R., Hall, M.D., Esselstyn, C., Jr. Reconstruction of the breast after mastectomy for cancer. *Plast. & Reconst. Surg.* 57:152, 1976.

Horton, C.E., Adamson, J.E., Mladick, R.A., Carraway, J.H. Simple mastectomy with immediate reconstruction. *Plast. & Reconst. Surg.* 53:42, 1974.

Hueston, J., McKenzie, G. Breast reconstruction after radical mastectomy. *Australian & New Zealand J. Surg.,* 39:367, 1970.

Hutter, R.U.P., Crile, G. Jr., Snyderman, R.K. The voice of polite dissent. Subcutaneous mastectomy for central tumors of the breast with immediate reconstruction. (Commentary) *Plast. & Reconst. Sug.* 51:445, 1973.

Imber, G., Schwager, R.G., Guthrie, R.H., Gray, G.F. Fibrous capsule formation after subcutaneous implantation of synthetic materials in experimental animals. *Plast. & Reconst. Surg.* 54:183, 1974.

Jacobs, E.W., Hoffman, S., Kirschner, P. Danese, C. Reconstruction of a large chest wall defect using greater omentum. *Arch. Surg.* 113:886, 1978.

Kleinschmidt, O. Uber Mamma-Plastic. *Zentralbl. f. Chir.* 11a:488, 1924.

Lilla, J.A., Vistnes, L.M. Long term study of reactions to various silicone breast implants in rabbits. *Plast. & Reconst. Surg.* 57:637, 1976.

McGraw, J.B., Dibbell, D.G., Carraway, J.H. Clinical definition of independent myocutaneous vascular territories. *Plast. & Reconst. Sug.* 60:341, 1977.

Millard, D.R. Breast Reconstruction after a radical mastectomy. *Plast. & Reconst. Surg.* 58:283, 1976.

Millard, D.R., Devine, J., Warren, W.D. Editorial on breast reconstruction: A plea for saving the uninvolved nipple. *Am. J. Surg.* 122:763, 1971.

Peacock, E.E. Biological basis for management of benign disease of the breast. The case against subcutaneous mastectomy. *Plast. & Reconst. Surg.* 55:14, 1975.

Pennisi, V.R., Capozzi, A., Walsh, J., Christensen, N. Obscure breast carcinoma encountered in subcutaneous mastectomies. *Plast. & Reconst. Surg.* 47:17, 1971.

Renneker, R., Cutler, M. Psychological problems of adjustment to cancer of the breast. *J.A.M.A.* 148:833, 1952.

Smith, J., Payne, W.S., Carney, J.A. Involvement of the nipple and areola in carcinoma of the breast. *Surg. Gynecol. Obstet.* 143:546, 1976.

Snyderman, R.K., Guthrie, R.H. Reconstruction of the female breast following radical mastectomy. *Plast. & Reconst. Surg.,* 47:565, 1971.

Snyderman, R.K. Subcutaneous mastectomy with immediate prosthetic reconstruction-an operation in search of patients. *Plast. & Reconst. Surg.* 53:582, 1974.

Spira, M. Subcutaneous mastectomy in the large ptotic breast. *Plast. & Reconst. Surg.* 59:200, 1977.

Verneuil, *Memoires de Chirurgie.* I. Paris, 1887.

CHAPTER 11

Medical Management Of Patients With Breast Carcinoma

BERNARD KABAKOW

INTRODUCTION

The medical management of patients with breast cancer encompasses both the initial workup and appraisal at the time of mastectomy as well as the workup and treatment at the time of discovery of metastatic disease. In the former situation, it is vitally important to identify the women who would be at great risk for tumor recurrence and more important whose survival would be shortened. It is hoped that the proper identification and treatment of such a subset will improve the prognosis. Treatment of women who initially are inoperable or who at some time following primary mastectomy have tumor recurrence is based upon many factors including age, hormonal status, and the sites and extent of disease.

PRINCIPLES OF CHEMOTHERAPY AS APPLIED TO BREAST CARCINOMA

The effectiveness of anti-cancer drugs is based upon their capacity to kill cancer cells before they kill normal cells. This selective toxicity is based upon a more rapid turnover of macromolecules, including DNA and RNA, in the cancer cell. However, because such normal tissues as bone marrow, hair, and gastrointestinal lining have the capacity for rapid growth, these tissues may be harmed by the chemotherapeutic agents, and the margin of safety, therefore, in the administration of these drugs may be a small one.

The chemotherapeutic drugs useful in the treatment of breast cancer may be divided into the following groups (Table I):

Table I.
Drugs Useful in the Treatment of Breast Cancer

Class	Dose and Route of Administration	Toxicity	Side Effects
Polyfunctional alkylating agents			
Nitrogen mustard	0.4 mg/kg IV q. 3 weeks	hematologic g-i local skin rash	may be instilled in pleural effusion
Chlorambucil	0.1-0.2 mg/kg/d po for 3-6 weeks, then maintenance (2-4 mg p.o. daily)	hematologic and g-i	
Melphalan	0.15 mg/kg/d.P.O. for 5 days, q. 6 weeks	hematologic and g-i	
Cyclophosphamide	40 mg/kg IV q 3 weeks; 2-4 mg/kg/d. for 10 days, then adjust for maintenance (50-100 mg/d.) P.O.	hematologic (leukopenia and anemia), g-i, hemorrhagic cystitis, and alopecia	
Thiotepa	0.2 mg/kg/d IV or IM/d. for 5 days, then adjust for maintenance (10-15 mg q. 1-2 weeks)	hematologic	
Antimetabolites			
Methotrexate	2.5-5 mg p.o. daily 0.4 mg/kg/d. IV or IM for 5 days, q 3 weeks 0.4 mg/kg IV or IM B.I.W. 1-3 gm in 4 hour infusion with Citrovorum factor rescue beginning at 24 hours	g-i (stomatitis, diarrhea, hepatic dysfunction) hematologic	contra-indicated in renal insufficiency
5-fluorouracil	12mg/kg/d IV for 3-5 days, q. 4 weeks 15 mg/kg IV weekly	g-i (nausea, stomatitis, diarrhea) hematologic	

Mitotic Inhibitors		
Vincristine	1.4 mg/m^{-2} IV weekly	alopecia occasional cerebellar ataxia
Vinblastine	0.1-0.2 mg/kg IV q. 1-2 weeks	neurologic (sensory, neuropathy, constipation etc.) leukopenia mild neurologic toxicity
Antibiotics		
Adriamycin	60-90 g/m^{-2} IV q. 3 weeks in single or 3 divided daily doses	g-i hematologic (nadir in 10-15 days), cardiac with total doses greater than 550 mg/m^{-2} alopecia
Mitomycin C	0.05 mg/kg/d. IV for 5 days q. 3 weeks 10-15 g/m^{-2} IV q. 5 weeks	g-i hematologic alopecia
Mithramycin	0.025 mg/kg IV q. 2 days	g-i hematologic coagulation defects hypocalcemia specific agent for hyper-calcemia

Hormones (see Table VII)

1) Polyfunctional alkylating agents. These drugs act primarily by inhibiting DNA and RNA replication by cross-linking the twin strands of DNA, thereby preventing the use of DNA as a template for RNA synthesis.

2) Antimetabolites. These compounds prevent nucleic acid synthesis, thereby inhibiting the formation of the purine and pyrimidine bases that are incorporated into the DNA and RNA molecules.

3) Mitotic Inhibitors. The plant alkaloids vinblastine and vincristine are derived from the root of the periwinkle plant and act by binding to the microtublar protein involved in spindle formation in metaphase.

4) Antitumor antibiotics. The various antibiotics useful in breast cancer treatment have different modes of action and different toxicities. Adriamycin, the principal antibiotic useful against breast cancer, acts by intercalation between base pairs of DNA, thereby inhibiting DNA-dependent RNA synthesis. Mitomycin C probably acts as an alkylating agent. Mithramycin, useful principally in the treatment of hypercalcemia, inhibits DNA-dependent RNA synthesis without affecting DNA synthesis per se.

5) Hormones. Androgens, estrogens, anti-estrogens, progestins, and corticosteroids all probably act by inhibiting the binding of nuclear and cytoplasmic receptors to the hormones.

It is presently thought that all mammalial cells, including cancer cells, go through a series of phases and that the above mentioned drugs act at different phases of the cell cycle (Fig. 1). Mitosis occurs in a very short period of time—probably less than 1 hour. After this the cell enters the first gap phase (G_1), a relatively quiescent phase whose duration is extremely variable. In fact, some of the cells may go into a stage of prolonged rest (G_0), when the cells are thought to be permanently non-proliferative. The period of DNA synthesis lasts from six to 10 hours and is followed by the second gap phase (G_2), which lasts approximately four hours and immediately precedes the mitotic phase. RNA synthesis occurs in both G_1 and G_2. The antimetabolites are cell-cycle specific, acting in the S phase, and kill cells in the active stage of cell division. The alkylating agents, on the other hand, are cell-cycle non-specific killing cells in all parts of the cell cycle regardless of the proliferative state.

METHODS AND PROBLEMS OF DRUG ADMINISTRATION, DRUG RESISTANCE AND IMMUNOSUPPRESSION

Drugs may be given by a variety of routes—oral, intramuscular, intravenous, or topical, or they may be injected directly into body cavities. Tumor masses devoid of a good blood supply are often resistant to systemically administered drugs. For the treatment of brain metastases there is only a limited number of drugs that can enter this area, either by

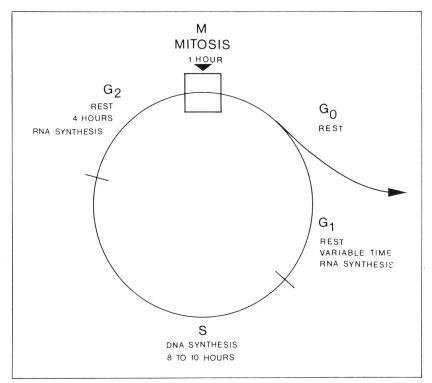

FIG.1 CELL CYCLE

virtue of passage through the blood-brain barrier or solubility in lipid (e.g., the nitrosoureas).

Knowledge of drug metabolism and of excretion is vitally important in treatment protocols. For example, cyclophosphamide is metabolized in the liver from an inactive to an active form and is therefore useless when administered into a body cavity. Methotrexate is excreted by the kidney in a soluble form when urinary pH is alkaline, and vincristine, which is excreted primarily in the bile, can cause early severe neurotoxicity if given to a patient with liver disease. Anti-tumor drugs may interact with each other as well as with non-cancer drugs, altering free drug levels and drug toxicity.

Finally, one of the great enigmas of cancer chemotherapy is the emergence of resistance to a drug that initially proved effective. The various cellular mechanisms involved in drug resistance include decreased cellular uptake, increased target enzyme, altered specificity of an inhibited enzyme, decreased drug activation, increased drug deactivation, increased DNA repair, and in some cases, development of alternative biochemical pathways that block an inhibited reaction. Many drugs given to cancer patients are immunosuppressive, and a few are even carcinogenic. Both of these factors have to be taken into account in the long-term administration of such agents.

APPROACH TO THE PATIENT AT THE TIME OF PRIMARY SURGERY

Whether the patient with primary operable breast cancer will be cured or not by surgery is really dependent upon whether the cancer has spread beyond the area operated upon. It is generally acknowledged that the goal of local radiotherapy is to prevent local recurrence. Two important considerations in future management are the presence or absence of hormonal receptors and the presence or absence of certain pathological factors and other considerations associated with a poor prognosis.

Hormone Receptors

Assays have been developed that can determine with a considerable degree of confidence which breast cancer patients will or will not respond to endocrine therapy (McGuire et al., 1977). This subclassification of tumors into hormone-dependent and autonomous categories is based on the presence or absence of specific receptors that are responsible for the binding between hormone and receptor protein and the effect of the latter complex upon the reproductive capacity of the cell.

The first such receptor protein to be studied was the estrogen receptor protein. In the hormone-dependent tumors, estrogen enters the cell and binds to a cytoplasmic protein receptor and this estrogen-receptor complex is translocated into the nucleus, where it binds to chromatin (Fig. 2). Other hormones with demonstrable cellular receptor sites include progesterone, androgen, and glucocorticoid. It is important to determine receptor status at the time of mastectomy mainly because when and if metastases occur, this study will serve as a guide to future management.

Historically, approximately 20% to 40% of breast cancer patients respond to some form of hormonal therapy, additive or ablative. Prior to the use of hormonal receptor assays, the decision to use such therapy was an empiric one. Now, however, such a decision is based on the results of studies of hormonal receptors done at the time of primary mastectomy. If estrogen receptors are present, the response to endocrine therapy is in the range of 55% to 68%; if absent, less than 10% (McGuire et al., 1977). More recent studies

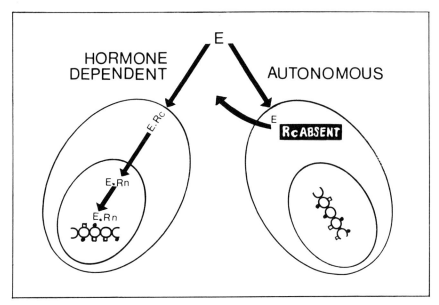

FIG.**2** ESTROGEN DEPENDENT AND AUTONOMOUS
BREAST CANCERS

have shown that if progesterone and glucocorticoid receptors are present in addition to estrogen receptors, then the response to endocrine therapy is even higher (Allegra et al., 1978).

Of all the prognostic factors studied at the time of primary mastectomy, the one most easily measured is the involvement of axillary lymph nodes and their quantification. The 10-year suvival rates are listed in Table II (Fisher et al., 1975a). In this regard, micrometastatic involvement of lymph nodes is of much less serious consequence than gross lymph node involvement; similarly, positive lower chain axillary nodes carry a better prognosis than involvement of the highest lymph nodes removed. Other prognostic variables that can be defined by the pathologist at the time of primary mastectomy are as follows (Fisher et al., 1975b).

Table II.
Influence of Nodal Status on Survival

Nodal Status	10-year survival (%)
Negative nodes	65
Positive nodes	25
1–3 nodes	38
4+ nodes	13
All patients	46

1) Histological grading. The more poorly differentiated the tumor, and the greater the frequency of mitosis, the worse the prognosis is likely to be.

2) Mucin content and tubule formation. In general, the more mucin present and the greater the degree of tubule formation, the better the prognosis will be.

3) Lack of microscopic circumscription. Patients with poorly circumscribed tumors have a worse prognosis than do those with well circumscribed tumors.

4) Associated proliferative fibrocystic disease. In general, proliferative fibrocystic disease in quadrants remote from the primary tumor signify a bad prognosis, whereas proliferative fibrocystic disease in the vicinity of the dominant mass have no adverse effect.

5) Tumors greater than 4 cm mean a prognosis poorer than that of smaller tumors.

6) Lymphatic extension, lymphatic vessel invasion, and perineural space invasion all indicate a poor prognosis. Blood vessel invasion by itself may not signify such a poor outlook, but when associated with other poor prognostic factors the prognosis is poor.

7) Invovement of the skin overlying the tumor, particularly its lymphatics, and nipple involvement both carry a poor prognosis.

8) Sinus histiocytosis and lymphatic infiltration when present make for a better prognosis, possibly indicating good patient immunity.

Some of the non-pathological factors that can influence prognosis are the following:

1) A long interval (six or more months from the time of discovery of the tumor mass to surgical intervention) usually makes for a poor prognosis.

2) Black women, particularly in the younger age groups, with large tumors tend to do poorly.

3) Women who are pregnant or who have had recent hormonal stimulation carry a relatively poor prognosis.

4) The absence of estrogen receptors in the original mastectomy specimen indicates a greater risk of recurrence and decreased survival, regardless of nodal status.

ADJUVANT CHEMOTHERAPY

The fact that the overall survival rate of patients with breast cancer has not improved over the last several decades has led to the early employment of adjuvant cehmotherapy following mastectomy. The failure of more radical surgical procedures combined with the addition of postoperative radiotherapy, to improve survival implies that microscopic tumor, incapable of early clinical detection, is present at distant critical sites such as the lungs, bones, liver, and brain. It is with the hope of destroying such distant micrometastases that adjuvant chemotherapy protocols have been devised. The principles forming the basis for adjuvant therapy are as follows:

1) The greater the tumor cell burden, the poorer the response to any treatment will be. The converse of this is also true. The less the tumor burden, the greater the chance of responding to treatment will be.

2) Because human breast cancer has a relatively slow doubling time, low growth fraction, and long cell-cycle transit time, treatment probably should be prolonged.

3) Intermittent therapy is probably better than continuous treatment because it allows for a period of marrow recovery, it may not be as immunosuppressive, and it may even promote immunological rebound.

4) Combination chemotherapy is safe and more effective in killing tumor cells than are single agents.

Current studies utilizing these principles include those sponsored by the National Surgical Adjuvant Breast Project (NSABP), (Fisher et al., 1977), the studies of the National Cancer Institute of Milan (Bonadonna et al., 1977), and those of Dr. Richard Cooper (Cooper, 1976). The NSABP began in September 1972 with a study of L-phyenylalanine mustard (L-PAM), or melphalen, comparing this agent with a placebo in women having had a radical mastectomy for potentially curable breast cancer and having one or more axillary nodes proved histologically to contain tumor. The drug was administered orally in doses of 0.15 mg per kg per day for five days every six weeks for a period of two years. Aside from mild nausea and some blood count depression, this regime produced no side effects. The results of this initial study showed a significantly decreased recurrence of cancer only in the premenopausal women, but no effect on the postmenopausal women.

The second NSABP study compared L-PAM plus 5 fluorouracil (5 FU) with L-PAM alone. Early results of this study show a slight trend in favor of the two-drug regime for decreasing tumor recurrence in premenopausal women. The Milan group has compared women with positive nodes found at the time of radical mastectomy who were either treated with cytoxan, methotrexate, and fluorouracil in monthly courses for 12 months (Table III-CMF) or who served as controls. At the four-year point, the overall relapse rate was 52.5% in the control subjects and 33.1% in the treated patients. When broken down into premenopausal and postmenopausal patients, the improvement with treatment was seen to be statistically significant only in the premenopausal group. Cooper, employing a five-drug regime (Table III-CMFVP) given for nine months post-mastectomy, has shown an improvement in the treated patients, both pre- and postmenopausal.

Table III.

Selected Combination Chemotherapy Programs in Breast Cancer
Presently in Use

1. AP
Adriamycin	75 mg/m^{-2} IV d.1, repeat q. 3 weeks
Vincristine	1.4 mg/m $^{-2}$ IV d.1, and 8 q. 3 weeks

2. AC
Adriamycin	40 mg/m^{-2} IV d.1, repeat q. 3 weeks
Cyclophosphamide	200 mg/m^{-2} p.o. d. 3-6, repeat q. 3 weeks

3. CMFVP
Cyclophosphamide	2.5 mg/kg/d. p.o.
Methotrexate	0.75 mg/kg week IV
Fluorouracil	12 mg/kg/d. x 4, then 500 mg IV weekly
Vincristine	0.025 mg/kg week IV
Prednisone	0.75 mg/kg/d. p.o., then taper

4. CFP
Cyclophosphamide	4 mg/kg IV d.1-5 q. 28 days
Fluorouracil	8 mg/kg IV d.1-5 q. 28 days
Prednisone	30 mg p.o. d.1-14, then taper to 10mg/d.

5. CMF
Cyclophosphamide	100 mg/m^{-2} p.o. d.1-14 repeat q. 28 days
Methotrexate	40 mg/m^{-2} IV d.1 and 8 repeat q. 28 days
Fluorouracil	600 mg/m^{-2} IV d.1 and 8 repeat q. 28 days

6. VACM with Rescue
Vincristine	1 mg IV d.1 q. 3 weeks
Adriamycin	50 mg/m^{-2} IV d.1 q. 3 weeks
Cyclophosphamide	100 mg/m^{-2} p.o. d.1-8 q. 3 weeks
Methotrexate	200 mg. IV by 3 hour infusion d.8 q. 3 weeks
Citrovorum factor rescue	15 mg IV 12, 18 and 24 hours d.8 after methotrexate q. 3 weeks

Adjunctive chemotherapy is not without side effects, and these are listed in Table IV for the CMF series. The question has arisen as to whether the beneficial effects in premenopausal women are due to drug induced ovarian failure. This has been studied by Rose et al. (1977) who found that after six months of treatment there was a sharp drop in plasma estrogens with a corresponding rise in gonadotropins. In the CMF series the recurrence rate is lower in those women having drug induced amenorrhea, but this has not reached statistical significance.

Other questions concerning adjuvant chemotherapy are:

1) Whom to treat? We believe in treating the subset of patients at greatest risk for recurrence and decreased survival—namely, those having a number of poor prognostic features present at the time of mastectomy (see above). Nodal status should not be the sole determinant of treatment. For example,

Table IV.
Side Effects of Adjunctive Chemotherapy (CMF)

	Percent of Patients
Leukopenia	
3,900–2,500	71
< 2,500	7
Thrombocytopenia	
129,000–75,000	60
< 75,000	19
Oral Mucositis	19
Conjunctivitis	32
Alopecia	69
Cystitis	30
Amenorrhea (total)	78
< 40 yr.	58
< 40 yr.	89
No toxicity	2
Failure to complete treatment	11
Drug-induced second neoplasm	0

the prognosis for a patient with a > 4 cm lesion with negative lymph nodes is worse than that for a patient with a 1 cm lesion with the lowest lymph node being involved. Similarly, 35% of patients with negative nodes are dead of cancer at 10 years after surgery and retrospectively, must have had distant microscopic cancer at the time of surgery. Detection of risk factors in this subset of patient and early adjunctive chemotherapy might improve the prognosis.

2) When to treat? Our policy is to begin treatment from 10 days to three weeks following surgery.

3) How long to treat? In premenopausal women, nine months of the CMFVP regime or 12 months of CMF seems adequate. In postmenopausal women, in whom the doubling time of the tumor is longer, perhaps longer periods of treatment would be indicated. In those women in whom dose reduction is necessary because of hematological or other side effects, we feel prolonged treatment is indicated to achieve the total projected cumulative dose.

4) The best method of treatment. At the present time, we are employing CMF for one year in premenopausal women, and the CMFVP regime for nine months in postmenopausal women.

5) Should adjunctive chemotherapy be combined with post operative radiotherapy? The latter has been known to decrease local recurrence, but is not generally acknowledged to have improved survival. Radiotherapy (Lewis and Paterson, 1976) has been reported to cause leukopenia in a sig-

nificant number of patients, and this would necessarily reduce the dose of concommitantly or subsequently administered chemotherapy. Bonadonna et al. (1978) have reported the local relapse rate in patients treated by radical mastectomy alone 15.5%, by radical mastectomy plus postoperative radiotherapy as 6.9% and by radical mastectomy followed by CMF, 7.2%. The conclusions from these studies would seem to be that chemotherapy might accomplish what radiotherapy does in preventing local recurrence, and without further bone marrow depression. The validity of these conclusions has yet to be proven by careful, controlled studies.

6) Are there any long-term harmful effects of chemotherapy? The potential dangers of adjunctive chemothcrapy, in terms of possible immunosuppression, carinogenesis, and myelosuppression, have been pointed out by Costanza (1975). Thus far, an increased number of second malignancies has not been found in treated patients, but such an increase has been reported when chemotherapy, used with other drugs, has been administered for prolonged periods (Lerner 1978). Finally, because 25% of patients with positive axillary nodes survive, disease free, for 10 years, and are presumably cured, we may be treating this subset of patients unnecessarily with potentially dangerous drugs.

A summary of the approach to the patient at the time of mastectomy is given in Figure 3.

APPROACH TO TREATING THE PATIENT WITH METASTATIC BREAST CANCER

The present management of patients with metastatic breast carcinoma, (Figs. 4 and 5) is determined primarily by the presence or absence of hormonal receptors. In the premenopausal woman with metastatic carcinoma, the chances of responding to oophorectomy would by 60% to 70% if estrogen-receptors are present and even higher if progesterone-receptors are also present. The reason (Fazekas et al., 1978) some ER-positive patients fail to respond to ablative procedures or to hormones may be a failure of the estradiol-ER complex to translocate into the nucleus (Fig. 2).

If estrogen-receptors are absent, then response to oophorectomy would be approximately 5%. In such cases, chemotherapy, using combinations of drugs, would be indicated. Chemotherapy very often ablates ovarian function, so that the 5% of ER-negative patients who would have responded to surgical castration would in effect have a therapeutic "chemical" castration.

There is a distinct advantage to placing patients who have had oophorectomies on adjunctive chemotherapy, beginning three weeks after surgery and continuing until disease progression occurs (Ahmann et al., 1978). At

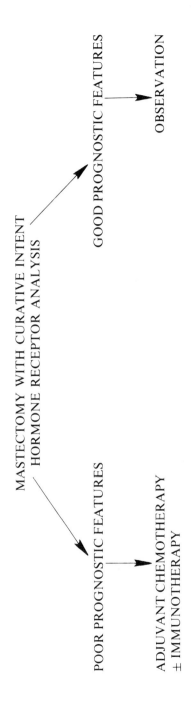

Fig. 3. Approach to the patient at the time of primary mastectomy.

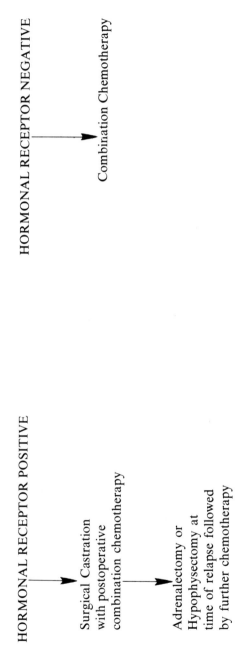

Fig. 4. Sequential treatment of premenopausal women with metastatic breast carcinoma.

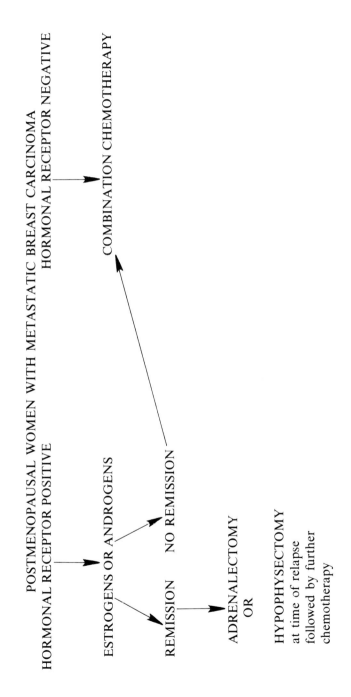

POSTMENOPAUSAL WOMEN WITH METASTATIC BREAST CARCINOMA

HORMONAL RECEPTOR POSITIVE

HORMONAL RECEPTOR NEGATIVE

ESTROGENS OR ANDROGENS

COMBINATION CHEMOTHERAPY

REMISSION   NO REMISSION

ADRENALECTOMY
OR

HYPOPHYSECTOMY
at time of relapse
followed by further
chemotherapy

Fig. 5. Sequential treatment of postmenopausal women with metastatic breast carcinoma.

that point, the ER-positive patients who have achieved remission with oophorectomy and adjunctive chemotherapy should have a further ablative procedure, either hypophysectomy or adrenalectomy. Results with both of these procedures are comparable (Table V), as reported in a national series in 1961 (MacDonald, 1978). Additional benefit from chemotherapy given after adrenalectomy has been reported by Wilson et al. (1971). Patients who have extensive liver metastases or brain metastases very rarely respond to adrenalectomy or hypophysectomy.

Postmenopausal women who had ER protein present at the time of mastectomy should be managed primarily with hormonal therapy, either estrogens or androgens. With increasing age, after the menopause (Hall, 1961) the chances of achieving remission with estrogens increase more than with androgens (Table VI). In addition, soft tissue lesions seem to respond better to estrogens, whereas, bony lesions seem to respond better to androgens. Overall response rates to these compounds are between 28% and 35% with a median remission duration of nine months. Progestins also have been reported to give remissions in breast carcinoma, though their activity is substantially less than ths aforementioned sex steroids (Ansfield et al., 1976).

Table V.
Comparison of Adrenalectomy and Hypophysectomy
in Disseminated Mammary Carcinoma

	Total cases	Postoperative deaths	Evaluable cases	Regression	Ablations to death (months)
Adrenalectomy	404	37 (9.1%)	315	100 (31.7%)	22.0
Hypophysectomy	467	42 (9.0%)	358	112 (31.3%)	20.6

Table VI.
Increasing Effectiveness of Steroid Therapy with Age

Age	Androgen-responders (%)	Estrogen-responders (%)
To 40 years	11	0
41–50	12	7
51–60	22	19
61–70	20	20
71–80	29	48

A new class of compounds, the anti-estrogens have been developed and one of them, tamoxifen, is beginning to be used more in clinical situations where estrogen-receptor protein has been demonstrated (Kiang et al., 1977).

The worst potential side effect of all of these compounds is hypercalcemia, particularly in patients with bone metastases (Hermmann et al., 1949). The clinician must follow the patient with serial determinations of serum calcium (weekly at first) and be alert to the development of the early clinical signs and symptoms of hypercalcemia—nausea, vomiting, constipation, drowsiness, and dehydration. Other side effects of hormonal therapy are upper gastrointenstinal discomfort (from stilbestrol), hirsutism (from androgens), skin rash (from tamoxifen), and fluid retention (from stilbestrol). A summary of the sex steroid compounds with dosages and side effects is given in Table VII.

Table VII.
Sex Steroids Useful in Breast Carcinoma

Class	Compound	Dose	Side Effects
Estrogens	Diethyl stilbesterol (DES)	5 mg p.o. t.i.d.	nausea
	Ethinyl		fluid retention
	estradiol (Estinyl)	3 mg p.o. daily	hypercalcemia
			feminization
			uterine bleeding
Progestins	Medroxyprogesterone		
	acetate (Depo-provera)	400 mg IM t.i.w.	occasional
	(Provera)	200-800 mg p.o. q.i.d.	hypercalcemia
	Megestrol acetate (Megace)	40 mg p.o. q.i.d.	
Androgens	Testosterone Propionate		
	(Oreton)	100 mg IM t.i.w.	masculinization
			hypercalcemia
	Fluoxymesterone		fluid retention
	(Haloestin)	10 mg p.o. b.i.d.	cholestatic
	Testolactone (Teslac)	100 mg IM t.i.w.	jaundice
	Calusterone (Methosarb)	200 mg p.o. daily	(Halotestin)
Anti-estrogens	Tamoxifen (Nolvadex)	10 mg p.o. b.i.d.	nausea
			rash
			hot flushes
			hypercalcemia
	Nafoxidine	60-180 mg p.o. daily	nausea
			alopecia
			ichthyosis
			phototoxicity
			hypercalcemia

CHEMOTHERAPY OF DISSEMINATED BREAST CANCER

Chemotherapy in the form cytotoxic agents administered singly or in combination, have been used in both the adjuvant and therapeutic management of breast cancer. The former has been dealt with previously. Response rates to individual drugs used in treating disseminated breast cancer are listed in Table VIII. Length of remission with individual drugs has, by and large, been short, usually several months and rarely more than one year.

By contrast, combination chemotherapy has produced both improved remission rates and increased lengths of remission. The basis for combinations of drugs (DeVita et al., 1975) in treating breast cancer is a biochemical one, aimed at blocking different loci or pathways in the synthesis of endproducts necessary for the growth of the cancer cell. As they have developed, however, drug combinations have evolved employing agents with different toxicities and also with different times after which toxicity would become manifest. The result hoped for was that the combination would give a better and longer remission than any of the individual drugs without producing overwhelming cumulative toxicity. Several such schemes are listed in Table III. In order to prevent resistance to any one combination, it is possible to employ alternating cycles of different combinations—e.g., two cycles of CMFVP alternating with two cycles of AV. Several of the combinations AV, (DeLena et al., 1975), AC, (Jones et al., 1975), CFP, (Ahmann et al., 1974) and CMF employ intermittent treatment schedules that enable a greater intensity of treatment to be applied and allow a period of time (one to two weeks) for the bone marrow to recover, and may also allow immunologic recovery of the host.

The disadvantage of such a program is that during the period of time when no drugs are given, rapid tumor growth of resistant cells may occur. CMFVP, (Cooper, 1969), one of the first combination programs devised,

Table VIII.
Single Drug Response Rates in Breast Cancer

Drug	Response (%)
Adriamycin	35
Nitrogen mustard	35
Cyclophosphamide	34
Methotrexate	34
Mitomycin	33
Phenylalanine	22
Vincristine	21
BCNU	21
5-fluorouracil	26

has the advantage of employing weekly intravenous doses of 5 fluorouracil, methotrexate, and vincristine, in addition to daily oral prednisone and cytoxan. Another program, VACM with Rescue, (Mattson et al., 1977) employs vincristine, adriamycin, and cyclophosphamide in the initial phase of treatment, and the relatively bone marrow-sparing methotrexate with citrovorum factor rescue in the latter treatment phase.

Certain cytotoxic drugs seem to preferentially attack specific sites of tumor involvement. Liver metastases respond best to 5 fluorouracil, bone metastases to cytoxan, skin involvement to methotrexate, lung metastases to adriamycin, and brain metastases to corticosteroids. With these considerations in mind, treatment plans can be adjusted according to the dominant site of metastatic involvement. In addition, drugs may have to be eliminated or their doses reduced in accordance with any organ impairment of the host. Cardiac disease limits the total dose of adriamycin, while liver impairment would lower any individual dose given. Methotrexate should not be given or its dose greatly limited with any impairment of renal function.

A comparison of responses to different treatment modalities is given in Table IX.

ROLE OF IMMUNOTHERAPY AND HYPERTHERMIA IN THE MANAGEMENT OF DISSEMINATED BREAST CANCER

In animal tumor models, particularly when the tumor cell burden is low, immunotherapy in several forms has proven beneficial. The application of various types of immunotherapy, either alone or added to chemotherapy, to women with disseminated breast cancer is still in an investigative stage. Results of studies to date fail to show enough clear-cut benefit from immunotherapy to warrant its widespread use. Several uncontrolled studies have concluded that the addition of BCG to chemotherapy may lengthen the duration of remission. In addition, the injection of BCG directly into a tumor

Table IX.
Response Rates to Various Modalities in Disseminated Breast Cancer

Modality	Response rate (%)	Time to response (weeks)	Mean duation of response (months)
Hormone additive-ER positive	60	6–8	12
Hormone ablative-ER positive	55	1–6	12
Single agent chemotherapy	20–35	4 or less	6
Combination chemotherapy	50–70	4 or less	6 +

nodule or in the adjacent skin can cause an inflammatory response with subsequent necrosis and disappearance of the local tumor.

The addition of hyperthermia to radiotherapy and chemotherapy may enhance the anti-tumor actions of these modalities. The hyperthermia may be either local or total body. Clinical studies are now being conducted to determine if hyperthermia actually will cause regression of breast cancer metastases.

REFERENCES

Ahmann, D.L., Bisel, H.S., Hahn, R.G. A Phase II Evaluation of Adriamycin as Treatment for Disseminated Breast cancer. *Proc. Am. Assoc. Cancer Res.* 15: 100, 1974 (Abstract).

Ahmann, D.L., O'Connell, M.J., Hahn, R.G., Bisel, H.F., Lee, R.A., Edmondson, J.H. An evaluation of early or delayed adjuvant chemotherapy in premenopausal patients with advanced breast cancer undergoing oophrectomy. *New Eng. J. Med.* 297: 356, 1978.

Allegra, J.C., Lippman, M.E., Thompson, E.B., Simon, R., Barlock, A., Green, L., Huff, K., Aitken, S., Do, M., Warren, R. Steroid hormone receptors in human breast cancer. *Proc. Am. Soc. Clin. Oncol.* 19: 336, 1978 (Abstract).

Ansfield, F.I., Davis, H.L. Jr., Ramirez, G. Further clinical studies with megestoid acetate in advanced breast cancer. *Cancer* 38: 53, 1976.

Bonadonna, G., Rossi, A., Valagussa, P., Ganfi, A., Veronesi, U. The CMF program for operable breast cancer with positive axillary nodes. *Cancer* 39: 2904, 1977.

Bonadonna, G., Valagussa, P., Rossi, A., Veronesi, U. Improvement of disease-free and overall survival by adjuvant CMF in Operable breast cancer. *Proc. Am. Assoc. Cancer Res.* 19:215, 1978 (Abstract).

Carter, Stephen, K. The chemical therapy of breast cancer. *Sem. in Oncol.* 1: 131, 1974.

Cooper, R. Combination chemotherapy in hormone resistant breast cancer. *Proc. Am. Assoc. Cancer Res.* 10: 15, 1969.

Cooper, R. Abstract in Symposium of Chemotherapy Foundation, Oct. 1976, New York.

Costanza, M.F. The problem of breast cancer prophylaxis. *New Eng. J. Med.* 293: 1095, 1975.

DeLena, M., Brombilla, C., Morabito, A., Bonadonna, G. Adriamycin plus Vincristine compared to and combined with Cyclophosphamide, Methotrexate and 5-Fluorouracil for advanced breast cancer. *Cancer* 35: 1108, 1975.

DeVita, V.T., Young, R.C., Canellos, G.C. Combination versus single agent chemotherapy: A review of the basis for selection of drug treatment of cancer. *Cancer* 35: 98, 1975.

Fazekas, A.G., MacFarlane. Nuclear estradiol receptors in human breast cancer tissue. *Proc. Am. Assoc. Cancer Res.* 19: 216, 1978.

Fisher, B., Slack, N., Katrych, D., Wolmark, N. Ten year follow-up results of patients with carcinoma of the breast in a co-operative clinical trial evaluating surgical adjuvant chemotherapy. *Surg. Gynecol. Obstet.* 140: 528, 1975.

Fisher, B. et al. L-Phenylalanine mustard (L-PAM) in the management of primary breast cancer. *Cancer* 39: 2883, 1977.

Fisher, E.R., Gregorio, R.M., Fisher, B. The pathology of invasive breast cancer. *Cancer* 36: 1, 1975.

Hall, T.C. The treatment of inoperable breast cancer. *Medical Science* 497, 1961.

Herrmann, J.B., Kirsten, E., Krakauer, J.S. Hypercalcemic syndrome associated with androgenic and estrogenic therapy. *J. Clin. End.* 9: 1, 1949.

Huvos, B.G., Hutter, R.V., Berg, J.W. Significance of axillary macrometastases and micrometastases in mammary cancer. *Ann. Surg.* 173: 44, 1971.

Jones, S.E., Durie, B.G.M., Salmon, S.E. Combination chemotherapy with adriamycin and cyclophosphamide for advanced breast cancer. *Cancer* 36: 90, 1975.

Kiang, D.T., Kennedy, B.J. Tamoxifen (Antiestrogen) therapy in advanced breast cancer. *Ann. Int. Med.* 87: 687, 1977.

Lerner, H.J. Acute myelogenous leukemia in patients receiving chlorambucil as long-term adjuvant chemotherapy for Stage II breast cancer. *Cancer Treat. Rep.* 62: 1135, 1978.

Lewis, C.L., Paterson, E. Leukopenia after postmastectomy irradiation. *J.A.M.A.* 235: 747, 1976.

MacDonald, I.A. Adrenalectomy and hypophysectomy in disseminated mammary carcinoma. *J.A.M.A.* 175: 787, 1978.

Mattson, W., Arurdi, A., Von Eyben, F., Lindholm, C.E. Phase II study of combined vincristine, adriamycin, cyclophosphamide and methotrexate with citrovorum factor rescue in metastatic breast cancer. *Ca. Treatment Rep.* 61: 1527, 1977.

McGuire, W.L., Horowitz, K.B., Pearson, O.H., Segaaloff, A. Current status of estrogen and progesterone receptors in breast cancer. *Cancer* 39: 2934, 1977.

Rose, D.P., Davis, T.E. Ovarian function in patients receiving adjuvant chemotherapy for breast cancer. *Lancet* 1: 1174, 1977.

Wilson, R.E., Piro, A.J., Aliapoulios, M.A. Treatment of metastatic breast cancer with a combination of adrenalectomy and 5-fluorouracil. *Prog. Rep. Cancer* 28: 962, 1971.

Index